# ACUPUNCTURE IN GYNAECOLOGY AND OBSTETRICS

*By the same author:*
ACUPUNCTURE ATLAS AND REFERENCE BOOK
ACUPUNCTURE TREATMENT OF MUSCULO-SKELETAL CONDITIONS
CELESTIAL STEMS
MOXIBUSTION (co-authored with Roger Newman Turner)
NON-MERIDIAL POINTS OF ACUPUNCTURE
SECONDARY VESSELS OF ACUPUNCTURE

A THORSONS COMPLEMENTARY MEDICAL TEXTBOOK

# ACUPUNCTURE IN GYNAECOLOGY AND OBSTETRICS

## *An essential guide for practitioners and students*

Royston Low Ph.D., N.D., D.O., M.R.N., F.B.Ac.A., Dr.Ac.

THORSONS PUBLISHING GROUP

First published 1990

To those many patients who had the courage to seek relief in alternative ways . . .

© Royston Low 1990

British Library Cataloguing in Publication Data
Low, Royston H.
Acupuncture in gynaecology and obstetrics.
I. Acupuncture
I. Title
615.8'92

ISBN 0-7225-2108-1

*Published by Thorsons Publishers Limited, Wellingborough, Northamptonshire, NN8 2RQ, England*

Printed in Great Britain by Butler & Tanner Limited, Frome Somerset

10  9  8  7  6  5  4  3  2  1

# CONTENTS

# PREFACE

As in my previous books, most of the material given herein is based upon lectures presented to the second and third year classes of the British College of Acupuncture. It would not be possible to give all that material, as in the absence of the necessary groundwork, much of the advanced teaching would be meaningless to a reader who has not previously encountered some of the premises. We hope, however, that enough has been included to enable the practitioner to build up a fairly comprehensive picture of his patient's condition, and thus to give a treatment based upon the soundest principles of both Western and Traditional Chinese Medicine.

# INTRODUCTION

For the practitioner of acupuncture, gynaecological conditions are definitely amongst the most interesting and, at the same time, most satisfactory he can treat. Interesting because of their variety and because of the thought required to discover their basic cause; satisfactory because of the manner in which they respond to the traditional Chinese approach once the correct diagnosis has been made.

As with so much of TCM (and I intend to use this abbreviation for 'Traditional Chinese Medicine' from now on), the diagnoses are based upon completely different premises from those of Western medicine, yet they are no less valid in their concepts. Western medicine is concerned with structural and hormonal changes, TCM is concerned with energic ones – with the movement of blood and energy – and a sound comprehension of both these concepts is essential if a true understanding of the patient's condition is to be arrived at.

In this book I do not intend to go into the basic anatomy of the reproductive organs – it is expected that the reader will already be fully familiar with this aspect. Rather, it is my aim to enable him or her to get a 'feeling' for what pathological or physiological changes may have taken place, why they have occurred and what, if anything, can be done to correct them.

As the frontiers of knowledge and understanding are slowly advancing, so a knowledge of the manner in which the acupuncture points perform their myriad functions is slowly developing, and we are only now beginning to realize their potency in stimulating the body's hormonal and chemical balance. That they aided the body in its basic objective of attaining homoeostasis had long been felt and speculated upon; that they achieved this via the stimulation of certain portions of the brain (especially the hypothalamus), plus a local bio-electrical stimulus causing biochemical changes, is one of the most fascinating discoveries of twentieth century medicine.

The thing which most intrigues me about gynaecology is that unlike most disease processes, where there is either an inflammation or a degeneration, or else an anti-bacterial or anti-viral response, in gynaecology we are frequently dealing with changes which take place within the patient's normal bodily milieu. These changes, as TCM shows us, represent movements in the fundamental energies of the body, impairment of which produce the various signs and symptoms embodied in the condition.

Western medicine lays emphasis upon the influence of the hypothalamus, the anterior pituitary and the ovaries in the production of oestrogen and progesterone to affect changes in the endometrium, thus governing the monthly menstrual cycle. TCM approaches from the view of various external or internal stimuli affecting the flow of Qi and Blood, and of basic Yin or Yang conditions.

As TCM is basically concerned with the accumulation and/or movement of energy, it

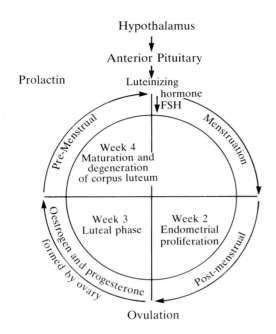

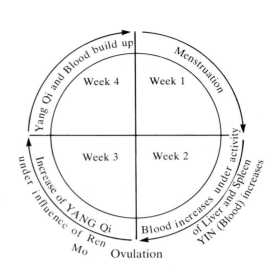

automatically follows that we have to consider the movement of energy in the body as a whole, and not simply in the pelvic basin. For this purpose the fundamental concepts of Yin and Yang have to be studied in greater detail than that usually applied.

The basic attributes are well-known to all:

| *YIN* | *YANG* |
|---|---|
| Coldness | Heat |
| Lower position | Upper position |
| Internal | External |
| Darkness | Brightness |
| Quiescence | Activity |
| Weakness | Vigour |
| Inhibition | Excitement |
| Slowness | Rapidity |
| Material, substance | Immaterial, non-substantial energy |
| Moisture | Dryness |
| Heaviness | Lightness |
| Conserves, sustains | Transforms |
| Contractive | Expansive |

whilst in the body, traditionally,

| *YIN* | *YANG* |
|---|---|
| Zang/Fu | Trunk and extremities |
| Chest, abdomen | Dorsal area |
| Below the waist | Above the waist |
| To the left | To the right |
| Body | Head |

| *YIN* | *YANG* |
|---|---|
| Internal surface of limbs | External surface of limbs |
| Internal portion of body: Zang/Fu | External portion of body: Skin Flesh Muscle |
| The Zang | The Fu |
| Blood and Body Fluids | Qi |
| Jing Qi (nutritive Qi) | Wei Qi |

It is stated that 'Yin is installed in the interior as the material foundation of Yang, whilst Yang remains on the exterior as the manifestation of the function of Yin' – in other words 'the Yin engenders the Yang' and Yang, the kinetic, depends upon Yin 'the potential' for its existence. And yet they are but two attributes of one and the same energy. There is no such thing as a Yin or a Yang energy – it is one energy functioning in either a Yin or a Yang manner. Hence the statement that they are interdependent and interconsuming; their qualities are relative and can only be thought of in relation to each other. An excess of Yang inevitably presupposes a relative decrease *in the Yin aspect*; an increase of Yin gives decreased Yang, a decreased Yin a false picture of Yang (because one cannot have a true increase of Yang if the Yin on which it depends is decreased . . .)

The relativity extends to all aspects. The head

10

is Yang relative to the abdomen, yet the lower part of the head is Yin relative to the vertex, whilst the upper part of the abdomen is Yang relative to the lower part and in the lower abdomen the right side is Yang relative to the left. These considerations need taking into account when we come to deal with energy movements.

One frequent source of confusion to students is concerned with the movement of Yang, as so many 'authorities' state that Yang tends to rise. So it does – that is its nature, its lightness, but that is its kinetic action as 'steam', and is against its normal flow. We have seen that Yang is predominantly in the upper part, and as far as its basic energy is concerned Yang tends to flow downwards. This is exemplified by the idea of the energies of Heaven flowing downwards to affect Earth and Man. Conversely, the energies of Yin flow upwards, and the perfect synthesis should be achieved in the region of what the Japanese call the Hara, just below the navel. The traditional statement is that Heaven affects Man and Man affects Heaven without affecting Earth, but Earth affects both Heaven and Man:

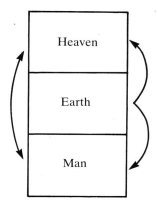

These concepts have their function in diagnosis and treatment when we come to the conclusion that, for instance, there is a stagnation of Yin in the lower abdomen. This means that there has been a blockage in the downward flow of the Yang, and the appropriate points must be chosen to remove this blockage and facilitate the flow.

# ACUPUNCTURE PHYSIOLOGY

In TCM the uterus is one of the 'extra-ordinary' or 'curious' organs, and is governed mainly by the ancestral energy, thus being dependent to a large extent upon the Eight Extra or Irregular vessels, and upon the metabolism of the ancestral energy by the Three Heaters.

Some authorities aver that both Ren Mai and Chong Mai originate in the uterus. Others claim that Ming Men (GV4) – the seat of ancestral energy – gives rise to a common trunk which passes via the uterus to CV1 (Huiyin) to give rise to Du Mai, Ren Mai and Chong Mai.

The Blood/Energy balance in the uterine (or pelvic) envelope is polarized by the envelope of the thorax, and both of these come under the jurisdiction of the Shao Yin (Ht/Ki) line, whilst the important irregular vessels are *Du Mai*, which supplies the Yang polarity as against the Yin polarity of Ren Mai and Chong Mai; *Ren Mai* – the 'Sea of Yin Meridians' – not only regulates the flow of energy in all the Yin meridians but is especially concerned with the Qi of the uterus; *Chong Mai* – the 'Sea of Blood' – supplies blood to the pelvic basin and regulates the Qi and blood in all twelve meridians; *Dai Mai* is the balance between the upper and the lower. The *Yinqiao Mai* helps remove stagnation of Qi and blood in the lower abdomen and functions at the level of the genitalia.

The Qiao Mai and the Wei Mai are concerned with different phases of the menstrual cycle (picturesquely referred to in Chinese as 'The Waters of Heaven') ruled by the moon – ovulation at full moon, menses at new moon, thus giving two phases in the cycle.

> Ren Mai rules the Energy,
> Chong Mai rules the Blood.
> Yinqiao moves the pelvic Yin.
> Yinwei balances the Yin of the lower abdomen.
> Dai Mai is used in pelvic troubles associated with loss of white fluid, etc.

So far as the ordinary meridians are involved, the important ones are:

Kidney: Is the basis of ancestral energy and supplies nutritive energy at the level of the uterus itself.

Liver: With Ren Mai, governs the smooth flowing of Qi; with Chong Mai helps store the blood, and with Spleen helps to hold the blood in the vessels. The Liver meridian supplies the region of the Fallopian tubes, and its point Li9 (Yinbao) increases the circulation of Qi energy in the pelvic envelope. As it stores the blood, if it stores too much we get excess menstrual bleeding or irregularity; if it stores too little, then there is not enough blood for menstruation leading to scanty periods or amenorrhoea.

Spleen: Holds the blood in the vessels and supports the pelvic viscera. It irrigates the ovarian region, and Sp10 ('Sea of Blood') is important in the circulation of blood at this level.

Heart: Is, as mentioned earlier, the 'polarizer' to the Kidney. The effect of emotions on the Heart can affect the amount of blood available in circulation. With the Kidney, the Heart makes up the Jue Yin channel which is the last of the Yin channels and is, in Chinese cosmology, linked to the lunar cycles.

By virtue of its close association with both Liver and Dai Mai, the Gall Bladder meridian may also be involved whilst its partner in the Shao Yang, the Three Heater meridian, also has connections with the pelvis and plays an integral part.

The principal meridians have their main connections:

Ki – via CV3 (Zhongji), CV4 (Guanyuan), and particularly Chong Mai.

Li – via CV2 (Qugu), CV3 and CV4.

Sp – via CV3 and CV4.

The Tendino-muscular meridians of the three Zu Yin lines have unions at CV3, where they also meet the Tendino-muscular meridian of the Stomach, which itself has a union with Chong Mai at St30 (Qichong). If the tendino-muscular meridians are out of balance they can affect the motoricity of the genital organs, i.e.:

Ki – can cause contractions and pains in the genitalia.

Li – is concerned with all pains generally, but has a special part to play in any motor imbalance, which can cause weakness. As an example, an attack of Heat can give a permanent erection, an attack of Cold retraction and loss of erection.

Sp – will cause 'pulling-pains' in the genitalia.

The Longitudinal Luo of the Liver commands all the genitalia, especially the vulva and clitoris via Li5 (Ligou), whilst the Stomach transverse Luo (St40 – Fenglong) by its connection with the Spleen helps to command the blood and can therefore help in haemorrhages and menstrual irregularity.

The role of the Distinct (or Divergent) meridians is not often considered, but it must be borne in mind that their union is deep in the body and in the head, and that the first couple, the Bladder and Kidney, pass through the Kidney; the second couple, Gall Bladder and Liver, pass in the pubic area, and the third couple, the Stomach and Spleen, pass at St30 (Qichong) which, as we have already seen, is

also a reunion point with Chong Mai.

When treating menstrual disorders we have to think of them in their relationship to the body as a whole. Acupuncture is concerned with the movement of energy, and this can take place in two planes – either up and down, or between internal and external.

The pelvis is the most Yin zone in the body, and if the Yang, which should go down, fails to descend, then it must be brought down, and the point we can use for this is St29 (Guilai) which is the point commanding the Yang in the pelvic basin. The point commanding the Yin, which should ascend, is Ki13 (Taixi).

The energy of blood and Qi should be distributed from the centre to the periphery and the point commanding this distribution is CV12 (Zhongwan). Distribution to the upper part of the body and to the arms, or to the lower part of the body and the legs, is under the control of the two San Li points – Co10 (Shousanli) and St36 (Zusanli) respectively. (Please note that the usual translation of San Li – 'Three Measurements' – is wrong. Li is indeed a unit of distance in China, but in older manuscripts it refers to aspects of universal energy, and San Li means the three transformations of energy, blood and air. The misunderstanding probably arose because Zusanli is indeed three cun below the popliteal flexure – but Co10, Shousanli, is only *two* cun below the transverse cubital crease, so the modern translation cannot possibly be correct!). A lack of central energy is possibly a more prevalent cause of prolapse than the more usually emphasized deficiency of Spleen although, of course, lack of Spleen energy will cause a lack of central energy.

The energy at the level of the pericardium is commanded by BL38 (Gaohuangshu) and at the level of the pelvis it is controlled by BL53 (Weiyang), the lower Ho point of the Three Heaters.

If there is a blockage of Yang in the upper part of the trunk then it is the Yang 'hinge', the Shao Yang, which is called into play, and we use TH12 (Xiaoluo) augmented with St39 (Xiajuxu) to bring it down. Yin must go up, and if there is an excess of Yin below we use the deepest of the Yin lines, the Shao Yin, with points Ki26 (Yuzhong) augmented by P5 (Jianshi).

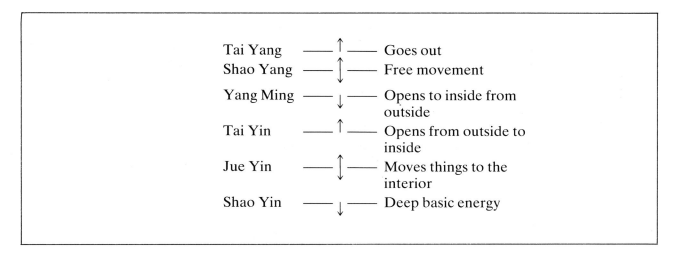

| Tai Yang | ↑ | Goes out |
| Shao Yang | ↕ | Free movement |
| Yang Ming | ↓ | Opens to inside from outside |
| Tai Yin | ↑ | Opens from outside to inside |
| Jue Yin | ↕ | Moves things to the interior |
| Shao Yin | ↓ | Deep basic energy |

If Dai Mai is too 'tight' it blocks the energy, giving stagnation of Yin below and Yang above, and we therefore open Dai Mai with GB26 (Daimai), GB41 (Foot-Linqi) and TH5 (Waiguan).

As a general overall reference for the movement of energy, the following points are extremely useful:

| GV14 (Dazhui) | Makes Yang go out and up. |
| CV22 (Tiantu) | Makes Yin go out and up. |
| GV3 (Yaoyangguan) | Makes Yang go out and down. |
| CV4 (Guanyuan) | Makes Yin go out and down. |

To bring Yang in, use St25 (Tianshu)
To bring Yin in, use CV3 (Zhongji)
To start Yang in general – GB25 (Jingmen)
To bring Yin out – GB24 (Riyue), augmented with GB23 (Zhejin)
To bring Yang out – CV17 (Shanzhong) (which brings it up to the Tai Yang level).

# DIAGNOSIS

The fundamental diagnosis is common to both Western and Chinese medicine and, as usual, starts off with the basic history – date of birth, married / single / widowed / divorced / separated, present and past occupations. The patient should then be asked the chief symptom of which she is complaining, how long she has had it, and how frequently it occurs. Emphasis will naturally be placed on the obstetric history – number of pregnancies with dates, were they normal (i.e. carried to full term) or was there any abnormality such as miscarriages, premature births, stillbirths or ectopic pregnancies.

Where the menses are concerned, we should enquire as to the patient's age when she first started and if there is any history of irregularity, the approximate duration of each period, and the number of days between the commencement of one until the commencement of the next. The amount and type of blood loss is important, and whether there has been any recent change. Dysmenorrhoea should be queried and its relation to the actual onset of bleeding, also any other associated symptoms such as headaches or nausea. Is there any other vaginal discharge, such as leucorrhoea? Is the discharge whitish or straw-coloured, mucoid or purulent or blood-stained? Has it an offensive odour, and does it cause irritation or soreness? What is its quantity?

Questions should be asked as to the state of micturition and the bowels. Is there any frequency? If so, does it occur during the day or night, and is there any pain on passing water? Incontinence may be of two types – stress incontinence which occurs on physical effort involving straining or, frequently, on coughing, or urge incontinence, which occurs when the urge to micturate cannot be immediately fulfilled. We should enquire into bowel regularity and whether there is constipation or diarrhoea, any history of haemorrhoids, or if the patient is using any purgatives.

The patient's marital history should be asked about, bearing in mind that many people sometimes find it embarrassing to discuss this aspect of their lives and that tact will therefore be required. The patient should be asked if she uses contraceptives and, if so, what type, also if there is any dyspareunia or difficulty with coitus.

The family history is important – the state of health or cause of death of both the parents and close relatives and the presence of any familial or hereditary condition. After this comes enquiry into any drugs taken and any treatment received. Any major illnesses or operations in the past must be noted and, especially in gynaecological cases, any current drugs used, such as tranquillizers, antibiotics, hormones, or the contraceptive pill. Has the patient been fitted with a coil, either now or at any time in the past?

The most important consideration of all is to ascertain whether there is any actual pathological condition present, and this will include carcinoma, uterine fibroids, patency of the Fallopian tubes or, looking deeper, a hormonal imbalance due possibly to pituitary pathology.

It is when we come to the actual physical examination that the traditional Chinese and the normal Western approach should overlap – both have much to tell us, but TCM frequently goes far deeper into what Western medicine examines only cursorily.

Traditionally, Chinese diagnosis consists of the four basic elements:

To look, to listen and smell, to ask, and to palpate.

## To look

This includes general appearance – short or tall, over- or under-weight, wasted. This is common to all systems of medicine, but TCM is looking for much more. A strong, robust type of patient is likely to have both a strong constitution and strong organs, and any imbalances are likely to be due to an excess condition. Contrarily, a frail, weak-looking patient is more likely to suffer from a deficiency state. Someone who is obese, possibly waterlogged or oedematous, is possibly suffering from a Kidney disharmony causing a deficiency of Qi, whilst a thin, dried-up type is more likely to suffer from a deficiency of Yin (causing a 'false Yang' which creates the dryness with deficiency of fluids) or a deficiency of blood.

The very way in which the patient enters the surgery is important – full of energy, outgoing, talkative is Yang; repressed, inward-looking, timid and cautious is obviously Yin.

The facial colouring is made much of in traditional scripts, invariably associated with the colourings attributed to the Five Phases:

Red     – Heart or Fire
Yellow  – Spleen or Earth
White   – Lungs or Metal
Black   – Kidneys or Water
Green   – Liver or Wood

This may seem very naive at first, but it is actually borne out to a certain extent in practice. What must be realized is that we are dealing with 'lustres' – a tendency or an underlying flush of a specific hue, and once that point is grasped then the correspondences do actually begin to make sense. A normal face

should be slightly shiny and moist, but a withered, dried-up look to the skin suggests a weakness in the vital processes which lead to a less favourable prognosis. The red face due to capillary dilation is well known and will obviously point to the possibility of cardiac involvement, but to the acupuncturist, mindful also of the 'atmospheric' correspondences, it will point also to a condition of Heat or Fire. Yellowness, in the west, would usually make one think of jaundice, with the Liver or Gall Bladder concerned, but for the Chinese it would indicate Dampness, more specifically by the Spleen failing to raise the 'pure' fluids. An 'orangy' type of yellowness, i.e. with a slight infiltration of the redness of Heat, would indicate Damp-Heat (a Yang condition), whilst a pale yellowness would be a Cold-Damp, which is Yin. The perennial question raised by students about the Liver and jaundice is answered quite simply by the fact that it is the Liver affecting the Spleen which produces the signs.

White is a sign of deficiency or cold. If the skin is dry and white (dryness = Metal and the Lungs control the fluids on the surface) there is a deficiency of blood. If pale, puffy and bloated there is a deficiency of Qi or Yang (the fluids are accumulating and the Qi fails to move them).

A dark blackish tinge is associated with the kidneys even in the West – the black rings around the eyes after a 'night out' showing the depletion of Jing energy, or the greyish tinge which appears after a long debilitating illness. The blackish tinge is always a bad omen, showing depletion of the basic Kidney energy, and invariably points to a poor prognosis.

The greenish tinge usually has a slight bluey or purplish touch about it, and is a sign of stagnation. The Liver is responsible for the movement of Qi and blood, and Liver dysfunction will lead to interference with this movement causing congealed blood or stagnant Qi.

### Tongue

An examination of the tongue comes under the heading of 'looking' and is, for the traditional practitioner, one of the most imporant cornerstones of diagnosis, but it should not be forgotten that the Western physician also examines the tongue, and when he does so he is looking for certain specific indications of specific conditions which must not be overlooked. The 'dirty, dry, brown tongue' of nephritis remains with me as a memory of my student days, and if I meet with one of these I am afraid that my mind invariably reverts to Western thinking, and I no longer think in terms of TCM tongue diagnosis but think instead 'This patient has nephritis – has it reached a stage where acupuncture can no longer help it, and is it a case for passing the patient over to those better fitted for dealing with a possibly serious condition?' The decision would naturally rest upon the performance of a number of tests of the kidney function which lie outside the scope of TCM as considered at the moment.

In certain anaemias (particularly pernicious anaemia and idiopathic hypochromic anaemias) the tongue may at first appear pale, smooth and translucent – one writer describes it as looking 'almost as if it had been boiled' – whilst in pernicious anaemia it may also be sore and develop into the smooth red 'beef-steak' tongue. The 'strawberry tongue' of scarlet fever is well-known – very red, with a slight fur and enlarged reddened papillae, whilst in typhoid fever the tongue is heavily coated, furred, and often covered with brownish sores. If the tongue is dry and the fur becomes 'caked' the condition may be grave, as it is especially indicative of serious abdominal disorders such as peritonitis or intestinal obstruction. Leukoplakia presents as firm, white indurated lesions but the so-called 'geographical tongue' is usually regarded as relatively harmless, being often a sign of a nervous condition or a mild hyperthyroidism. The tongue can change its appearance daily. Of interest is the 'scrotal tongue', so called because it presents grooves and markings very similar to those on the surface of the scrotum; it may be caused by a Vitamin B deficiency. In common with TCM, a small, dry tongue will point to dehydration.

The reader will thus see that although Western medicine pays some attention to the tongue, and some of its observations are extremely germane, it has by no means developed it into the art which has been achieved by the ancient Chinese, and an understanding of correct tongue diagnosis is essential for a proper assessment of the patient according to the Eight Principles.

In it, we are concerned with:
    (a) the body of the tongue, and
    (b) its coating.

*(a) The tongue proper* A normal tongue is of average size, light red or pink in colour, with a thin, white, clear coating. It is neither too dry nor too moist.

A very pale tongue indicates illness of the Xu or empty type, with a weakness of the Yang Qi, insufficiency of Qi or blood, or invasion of Cold.

A red tongue indicates either a 'hot' disease or a weakness of Yin from an internal condition.

A deep red tongue occurs in febrile conditions when heat has got into the interior of the body, or in patients after a prolonged illness where the body's fluids have been exhausted together with the deep Yin, causing a relative over-abundance of Yang.

A large pale flabby tongue, sometimes with toothmarks on the border, indicates emptiness of both Qi and Yang with retention of Phlegm-Damp in the interior (e.g. chronic enteritis). A flabby tongue which is deep red or with purplish-red mottling shows that there is an invasion of heat in the interior and excess Heart-Fire.

Some cracks or streaks on the tongue, provided there are no other symptoms of pathology, may be normal, but usually they indicate lack of body fluids due to an excess of Fire and a deficiency of Kidney Yin.

'Thorny tongue' is where the papillary buds are swollen and red, and indicate a pathogenic heat.

A stiff and tremulous tongue is often accompanied by speech and mental disorders, and indicates invasion of Heat from outside causing disturbance of the mind by Phlegm-Heat. Strong Heat can also damage the Liver Yin.

A deviated tongue shows obstruction of the collaterals by Wind-Phlegm.

Moisture indicates either unharmed fluids or the presence of Dampness.

Dryness indicates either harmed fluids or the presence of Dryness.

Thickness indicates severe vicious energies, a deep disease, or an excess disease.

Thinness indicates light vicious energies, a shallow disease, or a deficiency disease.

*(b) The coating* The formation of the coating is produced by the energy of the Spleen and Stomach which move upwards to gather together at the tongue.

Roughly, a white coating = a superficial, cold disease

a yellow coating = a deep, hot disease

a grey/black coating = a deep disease, with either extreme heat or extreme cold

but these are subject to variations according to the exogenic or endogenic perverse energy, and also to the stage of disease-penetration and the patient's ability to react.

A thin whitish coating can be normal. When Wind and Cold remain in the superficial regions, the coating will usually remain unchanged; as the perverse energy penetrates more deeply the coating will become thicker. When a thinnish coating becomes thicker and greasy it is usually a sign of invasion of the Lungs by Wind-Cold or by Phlegm (e.g. chronic bronchitis). A thick white coating is often a sign of food retention, a dry white coating of an infectious condition such as typhoid or some other plague.

As the vicious energies transform into heat the coating will become more and more yellow.

A thin yellow coating is usually an invasion of the Lungs by Wind-Heat; a thick yellow coating a chronic indigestion with accumulation of food in the stomach and bowels. As internal Damp and Heat accumulate the coating becomes stickier, so a greasy yellow coat indicates Damp-Heat in the interior, or blockage of the Lungs by Phlegm and Heat. A dry yellow coating shows accumulation of Heat in the stomach and intestines which damages the Yin (e.g. colonic infection).

When the vicious energy of Heat continues to move on into the deeper regions, the coating will change from yellow to black because it has caused harm to the nutritive energy and the Blood, which accounts for the fact that the colour of the tongue proper will be deep red gradually changing into a crimson tongue with a yellow-black coating.

If the blackish coating is moist it usually indicates excessive Cold due to weakness of Yang, or retention of Cold-Damp in the interior.

A dry, greyish/black coating shows that there has been a depletion of the body fluids due to excess of Heat (e.g. dehydration), or too much Fire due to deficiency of Yin.

Traditionally, the coating of the tongue is due to 'steaming up of the muddy energies', and, as we said earlier, must be correlated with other symptoms. A thick heavy coating is usually an excess condition, but it could be due to a deficiency of the pure energy allowing the Yang of Stomach and Spleen to 'steam up the muddy energy' and thus cause the coating. Inversely, a tongue with no coating could be normal, i.e. no vicious energy, but it could also be due to an absence of pure energy, which is thus too weak to 'steam up the muddy energy' and so form a coat.

Similarly where Dampness is concerned. If associated with Cold it can give rise to a white glossy coating; when tied up with Cold and indigestion, a white glossy greasy coat. If tied up with Heat, a yellow glossy coating.

As Damp can counteract the Heat which harms the body fluids, the coating may appear yellow yet relatively glossy and moist. However, if the Heat overcomes the Dampness the body fluids will be harmed and the tongue will become drier, yet feeling damp to the touch.

In the same way, a moist tongue may not necessarily indicate a Cold-Damp disease, because Heat energy may sometimes send steam upwards to cause coating; a dry coating is not necessarily a Dry-Hot disease, because sometimes Yang deficiency may cause an inability of the body to transform fluids.

Always we must pay attention to both the coating and to the tongue itself. Generally the tongue proper will show whether the organs, Qi, blood and fluids are Xu or Shi, whilst the coating will show the progress of the disease. If the coat changes from white to yellow to blackish the disease is deteriorating; if the yellow coating retreats and another thin coating appears, the disease is taking a good turn.

The 'peeling' coating, or 'Geographic tongue', or, if the entire coating peels off to leave a glossy tongue, is usually seen towards the end of a long serious illness, and indicates severe damage to the normal Qi and extreme deficiency of Yin.

(The practitioner should be careful to exclude such factors as changes in appearance produced by certain foods etc: e.g., a reddish tongue caused by drinking Ribena, staining from sweets such as wine gums, and the heavy fur produced by too much smoking or drinking.)

Finally, the tongue also has its zones, particular portions being affected by specific organs:

According to Henry Lu (translating from some of the oldest known manuscripts) the original divisions were as follows:

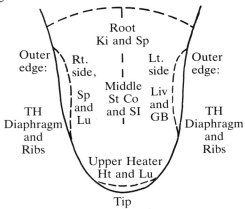

but later works give a slightly more simplified picture which appears to be more applicable in practice:

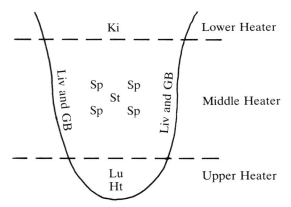

Examples of the application of this aspect would be:

> Heat in the Heart – tip of tongue red. If redness extends to cover a larger area, though, this would indicate Wind-Heat in the Lungs.

Indigestion in Stomach – middle region greasy.

Cold Xu in Kidney – Root glossy and white.

Damp-Heat in Liver and Gall Bladder – sides yellow and greasy.

Hidden Fire in the Three Heaters, or hidden Damp-Heat – outer edges deep red, although there may be a white coating.

Spleen Qi Xu – tongue normal, but both sides swollen and raised.

Liver Fire or Yang Shi – sides swollen, but *red* tongue.

The author has noticed in practice that a dirty yellowish-brown coating with a dark brownish root area is a sign of extreme malfunction of the lower heater as a whole. As a corollary to this, as the root represents the lower heater it will include the intestines and the bladder, and a greasy yellow coat will usually indicate Damp-Heat in the intestines or bladder.

Finally, some sources declare that the left side represents the Liver and the right side the Gall Bladder. To some extent there seems to be something in this, but as the tongue surface can also represent areas of the body –

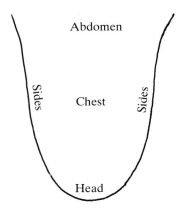

disturbance in the Ching Luo energy on the specific side must also be considered.

## Pulse

As with the tongue, the pulse is another aspect of diagnosis which Eastern medicine approaches in far greater detail than does the Western. Any practitioner, of whatever persuasion, will naturally take the pulse to ascertain its quality and its rate. The normal rates are usually given as:

| | |
|---|---|
| At birth | 130 per minute |
| In childhood | 90–140 per minute |
| Adults | 70–80 per minute |
| In the aged | 60–70 per minute |

but a trained athlete, because of greater development of the heart muscle, may have a slower than normal pulse. The Chinese were more logical in that, realizing the large variation from patient to patient, they assessed the pulse rate in relation to the patient's own respiration – four to five pulse beats to one complete respiratory cycle was regarded as normal, below that number was slow, six or more was fast.

For the Chinese, a rapid pulse indicated a Yang condition and generally a 'hot' disease, particularly in attack on the Fu viscera. Fast and forceful was a solid heat, fast and weak a deficient heat.

The West recognized the relationship between a rapid pulse and a feverish condition – indeed, the pulse rate usually bears a definite ratio to the height of the temperature, the rate being increased by an average of five beats for every one degree Farenheit (eight beats for every one degree Celsius).

Western medicine describes six types of pulse and two qualities:

| | |
|---|---|
| Intermittent: | Misses one or more beats (often sign of cardiac exhaustion) |
| Irregular: | Beats at irregular intervals |
| Dicrotic: | Excessive recoil wave (best seen on sphygmogram) |
| Pulsus Alternans: | Alternately weak and strong, though regular |
| Pulsus Bigeminus: | Beats occur in pairs, so that there is a longer interval after every two beats |
| Pulses Paradoxus: | Becomes weaker during inspiration |
| Soft | |
| Hard | |

A fast pulse rate – tachycardia– is found not only in feverish conditions but is also usually present in severe anaemias and will also be found following a severe haemorrhage. It is also one of the chief findings in Grave's disease (exophthalmic goitre), although here the pulse rate is out of all proportion to any concomitant rise in temperature. It is almost invariably present in cardiac failure and is important diagnostically in myocardial disease. Interestingly enough, to the best of my knowledge paroxysmal tachycardia is not described as such in any of the traditional Chinese literature – it is characterized by sudden transitions from normal rhythm to tachycardial rhythm and back again, and the paroxysms may vary in duration from a few minutes to even days or weeks. The stimuli producing the attacks can arise from the auricle, the ventricle, or the A/V node, and one of the commonest causes is disease of the thyroid gland.

A slow pulse (bradycardia) is most commonly from a heart block or aortic stenosis but is often common during convalescence from certain infectious diseases, especially influenza and pneumonia, whilst increased intracranial pressure with vagal stimulation (early basilar meningitis) will also produce it. For the Chinese it is a Yin pulse, and generally indicates a 'cold' disease with affection of a Zang organ attacked by Cold. A slow but forceful pulse indicates a cold accumulation into a 'solid' disease, but a slow and weak pulse implies a deficient Cold.

TCM actually recognizes twenty-eight different pulses, but there are twelve basic ones, the other sixteen all being variations on them. The twelve basic pulses, apart from the *Fast* and *Slow* pulses already mentioned, are:

*Superficial or Floating*: Felt on light pressure, becomes weak or disappears on heavier pressure. It is a Yang pulse and generally indicates superficial or external illness, or occasionally the onset of an acute disease. Floating and forceful indicates external fullness; floating without force indicates external deficiency or a state of general weakness and an emptiness of Yang.

*Deep or Sunken*: Felt only under heavy pressure. It is a Yin pulse, and is felt mostly in internal diseases of external origin. Sunken and forceful indicates internal 'solidness' and an accumulation of energy inside the body; sunken and weak indicates an internal deficiency and emptiness of energy. General deficiency states and respiratory disorders.

*Xu or Deficient*: Weak and forceless. Either disappears or is hollow and deficient on heavy pressure. Occurs in Xu type syndromes, with deficiency in energy and blood.

*Shi or 'Solid' (Excess)*: Forceful, even under deep pressure with big, rough form. Syndromes of Shi type disease, and extremely 'hot' symptoms such as high fever. Also hyperthyroidism.

*Wiry pulse*: Hard, tight, and forceful, like the strings of a guitar. Mostly felt in Liver diseases, where there is deficiency of liver Yin and excess of liver Yang.

*Rolling or Slippery pulse*: Smooth, flowing and forceful, 'like pearls rolling around a smooth plate'. Generally seen where the patient produces a lot of mucus, excessive phlegm or retention of food. May be seen in healthy people with ample Qi and Blood, and during pregnancy.

*Thready pulse*: Small and fine as a thread. Shows Xu (deficiency) of both Qi and Blood. General debility and also nutritional deficiency.

*Short pulse*: Movement is uneven and of short duration, with irregular missed beats. Short pulse of the Shi type indicates hyperactivity of Heat, excessive phlegm, stagnation of Qi and Blood and retention of food. Short pulse of the Xu type is a sign of collapse.

*Knotted pulse*: Slow and gradual with irregular missed beats, showing endogenous cold or retention of cold phlegm and stagnant blood in the interior. Deficiency of energy and blood, or blood clotting, or energy clotting and accumulated sputum etc.

*Intermittent pulse*: Slow and gradual, with *regular* missed beats. Impairment of Qi and Blood with declining Yang Qi.

Western medicine also recognizes combinations of pulse qualities, but again the emphasis is on the diagnosis of specific conditions rather than on the holistic approach. A typical example of this would be the slow, small hard pulse of aortic stenosis compared with the regular (but not feeble) pulse of mitral stenosis.

The size of the pulse is dependent upon the degree of filling of the artery during systole and of emptying during diastole, and is a measurement of the pulse pressure (the difference between systolic and diastolic pressures). According to Major 'The type of pulse wave which the palpating finger feels and which is more clearly shown in the sphygmogram depends upon the rapidity with which the pulse pressure changes. The term pulsus celer does not refer to the pulse rate inasmuch as it does not mean a rapid pulse, but a quick pulse, one which rises quickly and falls quickly.' A typical example of a pulse which both rises and falls quickly and is also very full and hard is the so-called Corrigan or 'water-hammer' pulse of aortic insufficiency. Note the Western emphasis upon using the pulse to diagnose mainly circulatory conditions, or diseases (such as hyperthyroidism) which affect the circulation, rather than the general state of the patient.

The difficulties attendant upon a correct assessment of the pulse according to TCM are admirably summed up by Dr Yves Requena in his book 'Terrains and Pathology in Acupuncture', (Paradigm Press, 1986) where he asserts

'In the description of when and how to take the pulse, many disagreements exist in China as well as in the West. Thus, Chinese pulse diagnosis never ceases to be a cause of argument for the layman and among acupuncturists. To the layman, it seems impossible to assess the health of the various bodily functions simply by feeling the radial pulses. Among acupuncturists, besides the internal disagreements about this diagnostic tool, some have rejected the concept of pulse diagnosis outright and do not accord it any credibility. Often their arguments bear weight. They refer to Qi Bo himself, who states, "The morning is the best time to take the pulse, as the Yin energy is sleeping and the Yang energy has not yet risen." Before the patient breaks his fast, the slightest perturbation is clearly perceptible. These practitioners argue that it is almost impossible, without a wide margin of error, to take the pulse at any other time of day. Let us imagine our first afternoon appointment, at around 2 pm. with a patient who has just had lunch and probably a cup of coffee as well.

Other acupuncturists think that without radial pulse diagnosis, there can be no good acupuncture. To soothe this argument, the least we can say is that pulse diagnosis is the most subjective aspect of Chinese medicine. It depends on the acupuncturist's values; it varies with the times of day, the seasons, the temperature, and it is not a scientific and objective means of diagnosis. Nevertheless, it occupies an important position in the traditional texts of acupuncture and the information gathered during its study must not be neglected. It might eventually help to correct an error of diagnosis. Thus, it is true that what constitutes the strength of a medical art may also be its weakness.

## To listen and smell

Listening in TCM means basically an assessment of the patient's voice and respiration. Just as a strong aggressive manner implies a Yang-type patient, so a strong forceful voice is Yang compared to a weak, hesitant, low voice. Coarse, strong respiration is a sign of excess, weakness or shortness of breath implies a deficiency. Wheezing is usually a sign of mucus. However, listening also includes auscultation, and the use of the stethoscope to ascertain any possible heart or lung troubles must not be disregarded.

Smelling is an aspect of diagnosis which used to play a far more important role than it does nowadays. The 'new-mown hay' smell of diabetes is well-known, but the mouse-like odour of typhus is equally diagnostic, and the urine-type odour emanating actually from the skin in certain rheumatoid arthritic patients is often very noticeable. Kaptchuk, in his book 'The Web that has no Weaver', describes two odours differentiated by the traditional Chinese physician – one, 'Foul, rotten, and nauseating, like the odour of rancid meat or rotten eggs', signifying Heat, the other 'less nauseating but more pungent or fishy, and may seem to hurt the nose. It is like the smell of fumes from bleach' and indicates Cold and deficiency.

## To ask

This has already been dealt with to a degree in the passage on history taking, but TCM enquires into various other aspects of the symptomatology, some of them very reminiscent of the type of details into which the homoeopathic physician would delve.

The 'Ten Traditional Askings' are:

(1) Chills and Fever
(2) Perspiration
(3) Head and Trunk
(4) Stools and Urine
(5) Food intake
(6) Chest
(7) Deafness
(8) Thirst
(9) Past History
(10) Causes

Some of these may not seem to be of immediate import when dealing with gynaecological disorders but actually, of course, anything at all pertaining to the patient's health and physical and mental make-up is of importance in arriving at an overall assessment. Whether the patient feels hot or cold, whether they *like* hot or cold, will tell us whether they are basically Yin or Yang, or suffer from a hot or a cold condition. If the patient likes to sleep lying straight out or curled up is not the sort of question the normal Western physician would ask, but again this would be indicative of a Yang or a Yin tendency respectively.

If the patient perspires, whether it occurs during the day or night is also important – daytime perspiration is a sign of deficient Yang or deficient Qi (the superficial Wei energy should be active during the day). Perspiration at night is a sign of deficient Yin. Medically, of course, it is indicative of tuberculosis.

The type of pain of which the patient complains will give us still further important clues. The description of pain is extremely subjective, but various types, locations and causes are traditionally described.

### a) Generalities

| Pain, | caused by |
|---|---|
| better for heat | Cold |
| better for cold | Heat |
| better for pressure | Deficiency |
| worse for pressure | Excess |
| better after eating | Deficiency |
| worse after eating | Excess |
| worse with humidity | Dampness |

| | | **d) Types of pain** | |
|---|---|---|---|
| with bloating or sense of fullness | Stagnant Qi | Stabbing pain | Mostly on the skin. |
| sharp, stabbing, usually fixed | Congealed blood | Burning pain | Mostly on the skin. |
| with sensation of heaviness | Dampness | Lacerating pain | Mostly in the muscles. |
| moving | Wind or Stagnant Qi | Dull pain | Mostly in the bones and marrow. |
| | | Aching pain | Mostly in the joints. |
| slight, with fatigue | Deficient Qi, or Dampness | Twitching pain | Mostly in the meridians. |
| | | Griping pain | Mostly in the internal organs. |
| | | Pecking pain | Mostly in the process of pustulation. |

## b) Causes of pain

**Heat** Skin flushed; burning pain; pain decreased when cold.

**Cold** Skin not flushed; no heat; aching pain; pain decreased when warm.

**Wind** Wandering pain with no fixed region, shifting around fast.

**Energy** Irregularity of attacks of pain; occasional twitching; prefers moving slowly, dislikes quick movement.

**Pus transformation** Acute and swollen conditions; no recess of pain; painful 'like being pecked by a chicken'; sensations of softness on pressure.

**Blood clots** Obscure pain at the beginning; light swelling; light fever; skin appearing dark brown gradually changing into blue, swollen and painful.

**Hollowness** Pain decreased on pressure.

## c) Attacks of pain

| | |
|---|---|
| Acute pain, sudden attack, sharp and severe pain. | Mostly in acute diseases. |
| Intermittent and irregular pain. | Mostly in diseases of the biliary tract, stomach, intestines, and parasites. |
| Continuous pain: i) No recess of pain, equal intensity. | In general symptoms of Yang diseases in their last stage. |
| ii) Mild and prolonged pain. | In general, beginning symptoms of Yin diseases. |

## e) Swelling with pain

| | |
|---|---|
| Swelling precedes pain | Shallow disease at the level of skin and muscles. |
| Pain precedes swelling | Deep disease in the tendons and bones. |
| Pain in several regions simultaneously with swelling or swelling following pain repeatedly. | Caused by current vicious energies or remaining poisons. |
| Wandering pain and dispersed swellings without formation of lumps | Caused by 'rheumatism'. |
| Extended swellings with pain in one fixed region. | Poisoning has gradually concentrated which seems dangerous, but is not really serious. |
| Extended swellings with pain in each and every part of the body. | Vicious energies have dispersed in four directions, which is beginning to pose a threat. Have a care for the future. |
| Swollen lumps as hard as stones, gradually increasing in size, causing twitching pain. | Very often symptoms of cancer and persistent chronic diseases. |
| Hard and large swellings: i) Already pustulated with pain | Mostly light diseases. |
| ii) Already pustulated, no pain. | Mostly severe diseases. |

### Urine and stools

These are considered by the Chinese in a similar way to that adopted in the West, but whereas the Western physician would subject them to microscopic analysis, the Chinese are more concerned with quantity and quality. Dark, concentrated urine is a sign of Heat and is Yang; copious clear urine is cold and is Yin. Concentrated urine which is accompanied by pain on passing would in the West lead to a query of cystitis – in China it would not be given a specific name, but would be regarded as a sign of Damp-Heat in the bladder. (Tests for albumin and sugar are, however, easy to carry out and should never be dispensed with, whilst if renal tract infection is suspected, it is always advisable to send a mid-stream specimen to a laboratory for culture and examination.)

Constipation with hard dry stools would show that excess heat was causing a drying-up of the fluids; diarrhoea and watery stools would point to a deficiency of Yang or excess Damp. Diarrhoea could also be due to the fact that the Spleen energy was descending instead of rising. So-called 'Summer Diarrhoea' – urgent, hot and burning – is a Yang condition; pale, watery, copious and gushing is Yin.

## To palpate

The final examination, palpation, includes the pulse, which has already been dealt with, and palpation of the abdomen itself. The general tone of the skin may also be included under this heading, and certain indications here are obvious – a generally cold skin will indicate a Yin condition and an absence of Yang, a hot skin the presence of Yang – either localized in the presence of a local inflammatory condition, or general in the presence of fever. In the latter condition, if the heat is felt mainly on light pressure, but disappears on palpating more deeply, then it is most likely to be the lungs which are affected; if strongest on medium pressure then it would be in the heart; and if the sensation of heat is apparent only, or most strikingly, on deep pressure, then it is possibly Damp-Heat affecting the bones and marrow. (The Ling Shu states that this palpation should be carried out on the anterior aspect of the forearm). A coarse, scaly skin is a sign of poor circulation of energy in the meridians, whilst if it is leathery and rough it is possible a severe lung problem.

When we come to the examination and palpation of the abdomen there are certain basic principles which should always be observed, the first of which is that before any examination of the abdomen or pelvis the patient should always be asked to empty her bladder. The first step is simply 'looking' – assess the amount of fat present; are there striae gravidarum from a previous pregnancy? Is there any distention or sign of a visible tumour? Next, test very lightly for any rigidity or sign of localized tenderness. Pain on slight pressure and a dislike of being touched are Yang symptoms, as is an increase in surface temperature, as we have seen. Pain which is felt only on deeper pressure is sometimes called Yin, but is really due to an emptiness of Yang.

The basic energy disturbances may be summarized as:

(a) Emptiness of Yin – Better for pressure and for cold, usually localized to the left.

(b) Emptiness of Yang – Better for pressure and for warmth, usually more on the right.

(c) Fullness of Yin – Worse for pressure, better for heat, usually more on the right.

(d) Fullness of Yang – Worse for pressure, better for cold, usually more on the left.

(e) Stagnation of Yin – Better for massage and heat, worse for cold.

Probing a little deeper, we next have two areas of exploration – firstly the abdominal areas themselves, and secondly the Front-Mu or Alarm points.

There are certain specific areas of the abdomen which reflect energic imbalances in the corresponding organs:

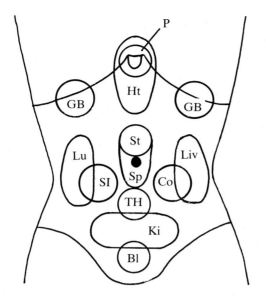

Students are always asking 'Why is the Liver placed on the left?' but, interestingly enough, if viewed from the posterior aspect the areas will be found to correspond to the basic '5-Element' or '5-Phase' pattern with the Earth in the centre:

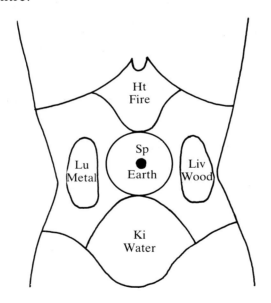

At the same time as palpating these areas for tenderness and temperature, attempt also to feel the quality of Qi in them, and also palpate the front Mu points. As a brief guideline, the Back-Shu points are used more for tonifying the Zang organs because they suffer from weakness, whilst the Front-Mu points are used more for the Fu which usually suffer from obstruction. Regardless of this, any increased tenderness over a specific Mu point will indicate a possible imbalance in that organ, whether Zang or Fu.

Next palpate down the length of the Conception vessel, or Ren Mai. Once again we are interested in the basic qualities – the temperature, dryness or moistness of the skin, elasticity of the skin, or if there are any palpitations present. On the thorax, if the skin is dry, lifeless and rough it is usually a sign of emptiness in the lungs. A very smooth and shiny skin is often found after apoplexy. If the thoracic wall is sunken over the points Lu1 (Zhongfu) and Lu2 (Yunmen) this also is a sign of emptiness in the lungs. The important points on Ren Mai are CV15 (Jiuwei), CV12 (Zhongwan) and CV6 (Qihai) but other points also have their indications. CV17 (Shanzhong) is the Alarm point of the Pericardium and also the Hui or influential point for respiration. It is the 'point that rules the energy' and, because of its function as the Mu point of Pericardium, some schools regard it as a diagnostic point for circulation. It is usually very painful where there is waterlogging and a hydrogenic constitution, but is also painful where there is atony of the stomach and in chronic and sub-acute gastritis. If there is pulsation at this point but not in the abdomen it is a grave sign – to be considered is the possibility of aneurysm of the thoracic aorta. This is almost invariably of syphilitic origin and will naturally have other diagnostic features.

CV14 (Juque) or 'Great Palace' is the Alarm point for the Heart. Pulsation palpable on gentle pressure is usually a sign of mental excitability – if felt only on deeper pressure it is indicative of a weakness in the heart. If there is resistance without pulsation then there is hypersecretion in the stomach, and if the resistance extends to the right hyperchondrium then the digestion is impaired and the emptying of the stomach is too slow.

CV13 (Shangwan) is a seldom used point but one which actually has many connections. If there is a wide resistance to pressure felt over this point there is usually a loss of appetite due to lack of acidity.

CV12 (Zhongwan) is the major point in Japanese abdominal diagnosis. It should generally be firmer than CV15 (Jiuwei) but less tight than CV6 (Qihai). If it feels like dough, soft and weak, and there is a noticeable pulsation, then there is atony of the stomach. If there is a deep-seated, root-like resistance, there is likely pyloric stenosis and hypertrophic gastritis. If the pulsation is very small like a grain of rice, or hard and stick-like, situated between CV12 (Zhongwan) and the navel, this would indicate emptiness of stomach and spleen. A strong aortic pulsation extending up to the sternum can indicate a psycho- and stomach neurosis, whilst a wide resistance on either side spreading to the sternum or navel indicates mental depression and insomnia. A stick-like induration extending from CV12 (Zhongwan) down to CV9 (Shuifen) can also indicate a pancreatic disturbance and too-slow emptying of the stomach.

CV9 (Shuifen) is the hydrogenoid point and the regulator of the water. It can speed up diuresis, and when sensitive indicates an imbalance on the elimination of water. If it is weak and lifeless, this would be indicative of a possible pancreatic and spleen insufficiency. A moderate pulsation is often present when there is general exhaustion and emptiness of liver and kidney; a strong pulsation occurs in the presence of psycho-neurosis, with the patient feeling unhappy and fearful.

CV8 (Qizhong) is sometimes regarded as the entry point of the life-force. If the navel is deep and well-shaped with strong surrounding tissues, this is traditionally regarded as a sign of strong resistance and a long life.

> If small, flat and shallow – insufficient vitality.
> If full pulsation around it – strong constitution.
> If the navel ring is weak – poor vitality.
> If navel and surrounding tissues dough-like – poor response and recovery.

If direct pressure to the navel causes antagonistic resistance, then there is emptiness of the kidney and especially the adrenal function. It can also be a sign of acute gynaecological troubles.

For the lower abdomen as a whole, if the muscles are rough and uneven, there is disharmony in the Three Heaters.

CV7 (Yinjiao) is actually the Alarm point for the Lower Heater, particularly its sexual aspect.

It is therefore a useful point to consider in all gynaecological problems.

CV6 (Qihai) is the 'Sea of Qi', and in health should be elastic yet flexible to the touch. If it should be soft and flaccid then the Qi is deficient due to basic kidney deficiency. If it feels tight on superficial pressure but becomes weak when palpating more deeply, there is excess Yang with a deficient Yin.

After palpation of the abdominal energies we now probe deeper still, and we are looking for definite signs of tumour or for any enlargement of the liver, spleen, kidneys, ovaries or uterus. Percussion will be necessary to map out the anatomical delineations, with succussion for the determination of any ascites which will also show up as a shifting dullness in the flanks with central resonance.

Examination will now proceed to the investigation of the pelvic basin, taking care to avoid any vaginal examination in unmarried women where the hymen is still intact – in this case examination must be performed per rectum, which still permits of bimanual examination.

Inspection of the vulva will show any swelling, ulceration or inflammation – the urethra is inspected for a caruncle or any urethritis. Oedema of the vulva may occur in some cases of nephritis or cardiac disease, but is more commonly the result of vulvitis or vaginitis. Pruritis vulvae, with marked reddening of the vulva, is frequently seen in uncontrolled diabetes mellitus.

Vaginal inspection is necessarily carried out with a speculum. The Sims' or 'duckbill' retracts the posterior vaginal wall and is used to inspect the cervix or anterior wall; a tubal speculum (Ferguson's) gives a good view of the cervix, whilst a bivalve speculum (Cusco's or Brewer's) can also be used. It makes for greater comfort if the instrument is warmed slightly before use.

With the possible exception of carcinoma of the breast, carcinoma of the cervix is the most common carcinoma seen. It usually occurs after the age of forty, is rare before the age of thirty, and causes three main symptoms: a watery discharge, often with a foul odour; bleeding, scanty at first but becoming more abundant later, and pain. Inspection will show either an area of ulceration or a bleeding fungating mass projecting into the vaginal wall. Although firm to the touch, it is irregular and friable on the surface, bleeding easily. Cervical palpation will also determine any softening as in pregnancy, or tears or polypi. These latter arise from the mucous membrane of the cervix, usually project outside the os uteri, are usually freely moveable and cause slight bleeding.

For bimanual examination the dorsal position is usually assumed, although some practitioners prefer the left lateral. The gloved forefinger is lightly greased and introduced gently to examine the cervix, and the other hand is now placed over the lower abdomen. By pressure downwards the uterus and adnexa are pressed down upon the examining finger and the uterus examined for position, size, shape, consistency, tenderness and mobility. In retroversion the uterus as a whole is turned backwards; in retroflexion the upper part of the uterus is bent back. The uterus may become very tender in inflammatory conditions, the mobility is affected by neoplasms and adhesions due to inflammation, whilst the size, shape and con-sistency are affected by neoplasms and (naturally!) pregnancy. The so-called 'frozen-pelvis', where the uterus is fixed and immovable, is usually the result of puerperal cellulitis.

In the normal way the tubes cannot be palpated under ordinary examination, but in diseased conditions bimanual palpation can indicate a prolapsed or cystic ovary, salpingitis, ovarian tumours, chronic pelvic inflammatory diseases with adhesions, tubal pregnancies and uterine fibromyomata.

The practitioner having explored the lateral fornices, the finger now passes posteriorly to the posterior fornix to look for any swelling in the Pouch of Douglas.

In cases of doubt, the patient should naturally be referred for further tests, of which the most widely used is laparoscopy, which allows inspection of the whole abdominal content, including uterus, tubes and ovaries. Ultrasonics are also becoming more and more widely used for diagnostic purposes.

# THE TCM APPROACH

As we have stated earlier, TCM ascribes all gynaecological problems to imbalance in the basic flow of Blood and Energy, and the causes of the imbalance refer us back to the familiar concept of the 'External and Internal Devils'.

The External Devils most involved are Cold, Humidity and Damp, the last two usually affecting the Spleen which governs the Blood.

The Internal Devils, which are probably the most important, would be:

**Emotional** Worry, grief, which affect the Shen or spirit, which affects the Heart to cause faulty circulation of the blood.

**Dietary** Poor food, imbalanced diet, which affects the Stomach/Spleen energy which affects the quality of Blood and Qi. (Note how patients on a 'crash' slimming diet suffer from amenorrhoea!)

**Over-work** Over-work and sexual abuse exhaust the ancestral energy and affect the Kidney Qi.

Any physical abnormalities which have developed are considered to be due to the involvement of one or more of these pernicious influences interacting upon the basic hereditary make-up of the patient and upon any predisposing factors which may be present. In all disease processes they pass first through a phase where the energy becomes imbalanced leading to a disturbance of function. Only where this remains uncorrected will an actual physical lesion occur. It therefore necessarily follows that as

practitioners our first priority is, if possible, to intervene during the energetic phase and to correct this. Structural anomalies developing from congenital or hereditary factors are usually considered to be outside our terms of reference, which is why it is so important to rule these out in our preliminary examination.

The two factors we are now concerned with are Energy and Blood, with weakness or stagnation of one or the other giving rise to various symptoms, though most troubles have their origin in the blood, which opposes the energy. The blood is a composite of liquids and solids, and the liquids in their turn are formed from Yin and Yang, or Matter and Energy. Yang makes the Yin circulate, and the Qi energy which is more Yang makes the Blood, which is more Yin, circulate. As we can see from our diagram 2 in the Introduction, the build-up of Yang pre-menstrually gives an increase of energy which pushes the matter, and it is this which causes the menses.

If the energy is in excess the blood circulates too quickly; if it increases even more the periods become full and of short duration; still more, and the blood is pushed so much as to escape from the vessels, to cause epistaxis and bleeding between the periods.

A deficiency of energy leads to stagnation and a shortening of the menstrual spacing, whilst a still greater deficiency leads to an actual escape of matter – a stagnant seepage rather than the 'pushing-out' caused by energetic excess. But all is relative, and most troubles are due to emptiness – either a general weakness of energy and blood which will produce abundant periods, weak energy which will produce very abundant periods and escape of vaginal fluids (leucorrhoea), or weak blood, which can lead to sterility.

The main types of gynaecological disorder considered by TCM are: amenorrhoea, dysmenorrhoea, irregular menses, abnormal uterine bleeding, leucorrhoea, endometriosis, premenstrual tension, menopausal symptoms, uterine displacements and infertility (both male and female), and we shall now consider them in detail. Also to be considered are disorders of pregnancy: morning sickness, abdominal pain, oedema, eclampsia gravidarum, vaginal bleeding, dysuria, abortion and miscarriage, to be followed by notes on the induction of labour and post-partum disorders: retention of the placenta, retention of lochia, lochiorrhoea, abdominal pain, fainting, fever, constipation, urinary incontinence, scanty lactation, and mastitis.

# Part One:
# Considerations in detail

# AMENORRHOEA

Amenorrhoea, or absence of menstruation, may be apparent or real. Apparent amenorrhoea (or cryptomenorrhoea) may have several causes. Occasionally it is met with in young girls who have experienced the monthly pains for a long time but have never menstruated – this may be due to an imperforate hymen or vaginal atresia, which would mean that the menstrual blood accumulates in the vagina yet is unable to escape. This build-up in the vagina sometimes causes a swelling which presses down on the bladder and causes retention of urine – so-called haematocolpos. In a long-standing case the clot may also fill the uterus (haematometra) or even the tubes (haematosalpynx). This condition will call for surgical intervention, with the performance of hymenectomy and the evacuation of the blood.

During the preliminary physical examination the practitioner will also have looked for such rare conditions as congenital absence of the vagina or uterus, or a short blind vagina such as can occur from testicular feminization.

Real amenorrhoea may be primary or secondary. Primary amenorrhoea means that menstruation has been delayed beyond the age of puberty. This is often not too serious, and it may be simply a case of late development, but if the girl is less than four feet ten inches in height by the age of sixteen there is the possibility of ovarian agenesis (Turner's syndrome) or panhypopituitarism, whilst if there are virilizing changes, the excretion of 17-oxosteroids will be increased in congenital or acquired adrenogenital syndrome. An adrenal tumour may be excluded by the dexamethasone suppression test.

Secondary amenorrhoea means that after normal menstruation has been established for a long period it suddenly ceases. The most obvious cause, of course, is pregnancy, but it can occur after any debilitating disease, especially pulmonary tuberculosis. Sometimes a drastic change of work or lifestyle or climate can bring it on, or a sudden mental shock, whilst starvation or severe slimming regimes (as in anorexia nervosa) may also cause it. It may also be caused by obesity, whilst it is a side-effect of some drugs such as digoxin, reserpine, phenothiazines and hormones (including oral contraceptives). An early menopause must naturally be taken into consideration.

From the point of view of TCM there are two main causes:

## Stagnant Blood

This gives an excess (Shi) condition. It is characterized by sudden onset, and is usually from mental depression causing the blood to coagulate and obstruct the channels and disrupt the functions of Chong Mai and Ren Mai, thus leading to stagnant Liver Qi. There can be distention of the breasts and flanks, with pain in the lower abdomen, worse with pressure. There may be abdominal lumps, whilst the skin tends

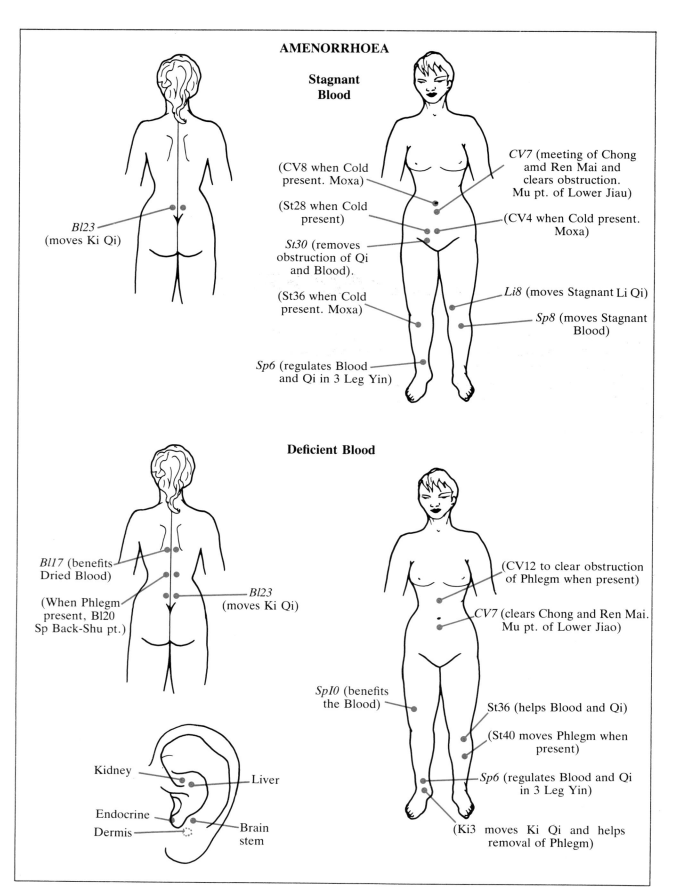

**AMENORRHOEA**

**Stagnant Blood**

*Bl23* (moves Ki Qi)

(CV8 when Cold present. Moxa)

(St28 when Cold present)

*St30* (removes obstruction of Qi and Blood).

(St36 when Cold present. Moxa)

*Sp6* (regulates Blood and Qi in 3 Leg Yin)

*CV7* (meeting of Chong amd Ren Mai and clears obstruction. Mu pt. of Lower Jiau)

(CV4 when Cold present. Moxa)

*Li8* (moves Stagnant Li Qi)

*Sp8* (moves Stagnant Blood)

**Deficient Blood**

*Bl17* (benefits Dried Blood)

(When Phlegm present, Bl20 Sp Back-Shu pt.)

*Bl23* (moves Ki Qi)

Kidney

Liver

Endocrine

Dermis

Brain stem

*Sp10* (benefits the Blood)

(CV12 to clear obstruction of Phlegm when present)

*CV7* (clears Chong and Ren Mai. Mu pt. of Lower Jiao)

St36 (helps Blood and Qi)

(St40 moves Phlegm when present)

*Sp6* (regulates Blood and Qi in 3 Leg Yin)

(Ki3 moves Ki Qi and helps removal of Phlegm)

to be scaly. In serious conditions the patient may be constipated. The tongue frequently has a sticky whitish coating, and the pulse tends to be thready and wiry. This type of amenorrhoea may also be caused by exposure to cold, which causes a stagnation of 'Evil Qi' in the womb. The patient will have a typical aversion to cold, possibly a stiffness in the neck and lumbar areas, whilst there may also be leucorrhoea. The tongue will be darkish and the pulse deep and hesitant or retarded.

## Deficient Blood

This is a deficient (Xu) condition. In this case the menses gradually diminish. It is common after a long illness causing depletion of Kidney Qi, after too many pregnancies, after anxiety causing weakening of Spleen and Stomach with exhaustion of the Yin blood. Chong Mai and Ren Mai will also be depleted. This condition, owing to the weakness in the blood, may present with a sallow complexion, dry skin, lassitude, weakness, night sweats, dizziness, palpitations, loose stools and loss of appetite. The tongue will have a whitish coat and the pulse will be weak and forceless.

A few cases of 'Blood Deficiency' type may be due to Obstruction of Phlegm, This will typically give a general 'puffy and stuffy' appearance, with distention, obesity, poor appetite, profuse sputum, and possibly leucorrhoea. The tongue coating will be white and sticky, the pulse slippery and wiry.

The treatment in both cases will be directed towards improving the Kidney Qi and to regulating Chong Mai and Ren Mai, also to helping the Spleen which, by its transforming function, will strengthen the Kidney Qi.

In both cases, the principal points chosen are:

BL23 (Shenshu) (Strengthens Kidney Qi)
CV7 (Yinjiao) (Meeting point of Chong Mai and Ren Mai and clears obstruction from them. It is also the Front-Mu point of the Lower Heater)
Sp6 (Sanyin jiao) (Regulates blood and Qi in the three leg Yin)

and one then adds:

In (a) Stagnant Blood:
SL30 (Qichong) (Meeting place of Stomach and Chong Mai. Removes obstruction of Qi and dispels coagulation of blood)
Sp8 (Diji) (Moves stagnant blood)
Li8 (Ququan) (Moves stagnant Liver Qi)
Alternative points chosen might be such as CV3 (Zhongji), Co4 (Hegu) or Li2 (Xingjian).

In cases of stagnant blood due to exposure to cold the emphasis will naturally be on the use of moxibustion to combat the cold, and the points added could be CV4 (Guanyuan), CV8 (Shenque – moxa on salt), St28 (Shuidao) and St36 (Zusanli).

(b) Deficient Blood:
Bl17 (Geshu) (Benefits 'dried' blood)
Sp10 (Xuehai) (Benefits the blood)
or, possibly, B120 (Pishu), St36 (Zusanli), CV6 (Qihai) and CV4 (Guanyuan).

In cases of obstruction of phlegm, we would add CV3 (Zhongji), CV12 (Zhongwan), St30 (Qichong), St40 (Fenglong), B120 (Pishu) and Ki3 (Taixi).

Typical auricular points used could be Endocrine, Kidney, Liver, Brain Stem and Dermis.

# DYSMENORRHOEA

Medically, this consists of three main types:
 (i) Spasmodic (Primary or Intrinsic)
 (ii) Congestive (Secondary or Acquired)
 (iii) Membranous

## Spasmodic

This is possibly the commonest type of dysmenorrhoea and is most usual in the younger, single woman, being in most cases worst between the ages of eighteen and thirty years, and there is frequently a history of acute pain dating from soon after or three to four years after the commencement of menstruation. The pain may be continuous but is frequently spasmodic and comes on during the early stages of the periods, and may be accompanied by sweating, headaches, vomiting and fainting. The pain is muscular in origin and is most likely caused by ischaemia due to contraction of the uterine muscles, and is felt in the low-back and pelvis, occasionally radiating into the legs. The attacks usually last from twelve to twenty-four hours. The condition frequently disappears after childbirth, possibly because of the increased vascularity of the uterus.

## Congestive

This type affects an older age group, usually women over thirty, being very rare before the age of twenty-five. The pain is of a less acute type and begins between three to seven days before the periods start. During this time the pelvic organs are always more congested with blood than is usual, and certain conditions will increase this congestion. The two principal ones are chronic pelvic sepsis and endometriosis, but malposition of the uterus or ovarian fibroids, or occasionally habitual constipation, may be causes.

The presenting symptoms are dull, aching pains in the low back and pelvis, headache, and a sensation of heaviness and fullness, made worse by exertion. They usually disappear when the menstrual flow begins, but are occasionally exacerbated.

## Membranous

This is a very rare and painful condition where the whole of the endometrium is shed at once, rather than coming away piecemeal. It may occur at every period, or only occasionally, but the pain ceases once the cast is passed. Sometimes the symptoms are similar to those of spasmodic dysmenorrhoea, and this can occur when large fragments of the endometrium are passed.

Acupuncture is of no use where the causes are organic infection, lesions, or some irreversible condition. In these instances the patient should necessarily be referred to a consultant, but dysmenorrhoea due to endometriosis, pelvic inflammatory disease, even uterine ante- or retroversion are all treatable by TCM, the first two usually being regarded as being due to retardation of Qi and stagnation of blood.

As in all cases of diagnosis through the aspects of TCM, we are concerned with determining whether the condition is of an internal or an external origin, whether it is due to an excess or a deficiency, and whether it is due to a basically Yin or Yang imbalance.

An external cause will usually be due to the influence of cold on the cycle, either from atmospheric cold or even the imbibing of too many cold drinks; the internal causes could be due to faulty diet or, frequently, the result of mental unrest. The resulting pathology will be either a disturbance on the general movement of the energy of Qi and blood, or a quantitive imbalance between Yin and Yang. As with most gynaecological conditions, the channels most intimately concerned are Ren Mai, Chong Mai, the Liver and Spleen meridians, and possibly Dai Mai as the 'belt' between upper and lower aspects. The Kidney channel will play an important role where the state of the Yuan Qi comes into question.

In diagnosis, the question of time is of paramount importance – does the pain first come on before, during, or after the menses? Further questions concern the *quality* of the pain – is it sharp or stabbing, or a dull, distended ache? Is it made worse or better by pressure, is it made worse by the application of heat or cold? Is there abdominal distention? Does the pain appear more to the left or to the right of the abdomen? Despite the traditional affirmations that the left side of the body is Yang and the right side Yin, remembering our earlier statements about Yang tending to go to the right and Yin to the left the answer to the final question will give us an important clue as to whether we are dealing with a Yin or a Yang imbalance, having regard to the fact that in a pathological condition this movement will be impeded and the symptoms will appear on the opposite side, thus:

### (a) Fullness of Yang
Usually on the left, worse for pressure, better for cold. Spasms and sensations of heat in lower abdomen.

*Treatment*: Get the Yang moving via the barrier point B129 (Zhonglushu), then help it to rise by the use of GV20 (Baihui) and Sp6 (Sanyinjiao). If the Yin is not 'blocked' inside, use Ki15 (Zhongzhu) to pass the Yin to the interior, and Ki4 (Dazhong) which passes the energy from the exterior to the interior.

### (b) Fullness of Yin
Usually on the right, worse for pressure, better for heat. Spasmodic pains appearing well before the menses, during the most Yin part of the cycle, before the Yang has a chance to build. Often with constipation and polyuria.

*Treatment*: If Yin is blocked in the pelvis and fails to rise, use the barrier point Ki18 (Shiguan) followed by CV4 (Guanyuan) to get the Yin moving.

To increase the circulation of Yin, Ki26 (Yuzhong) and Ki13 (Qixue), also Sp13 (Fushe), which moves the Yin of the trunk.

If the Yang is not 'blocked' inside, St25 (Tianshu) makes the Yang go in, whilst St40 (Fenglong) sends the Yang energy from the exterior to the interior.

### (c) Emptiness of Yang
Usually more to the right, better for pressure and warmth. Dull continuous pain, often with colitis or cystitis.

*Treatment*: If there is a general lack of Yang with excess of Yin (pulses usually full on the right and deficient on the left) then tonify the Spleen – B120 (Pishu), Sp2 (Dadu), Sp3 (Taibai), Sp9 (Yinlingquan) and Lu9 (Taiyuan), and mobilize the Shao Yang via B134 (Xialiao) and TH5 (Waiguan).

If the condition is a *local* excess of Yin in the pelvis, thus blocking the entrance of Yang and causing a passive congestion, then mobilize the Yin and bring the Yang in – Moxa B131 (Shangliao), B135 (Huiyang), GV4 (Mingmen), B123 (Shenshu); open Dai Mai – GB41 (Lingqi), GB26 (Daimai); mobilize Jueh Yin channel by the Yong and Yu points Li2 (Xingjian), Li3 (Taichong) and P5 (Jianshi) and P6 (Neiguan).

### (d) Emptiness of Yin
Usually more to the left, better for pressure and cold. Presents with Yang symptoms of spasm and pre-menstrual distention.

*Treatment*: Bring Yin in via Ki15 (Zhongshu) and Ki4 (Dazhong).

**(e) Stagnation of Yin**
Usually central, better for massage and heat, worse for cold. Often accompanied by diarrhoea, or constipation; cystitis; delayed digestion.

*Treatment*: Move the Yin – Moxa CV4 (Guanyuan), Sp6 (Sanyinjiao), Sp10 (Xuehai), also GV4 (Mingmen) and B123 (Shenshu) to move the Yang.

In the above conditions we are approaching purely from the aspect of energy movement, and disregarding the more usual 'Eight Principle' viewpoint. It will be found, however, that such a simplified approach as the one given can often prove enormously effective and is well worth while considering. The practitioner should always be recognizant of the fact that pain occurring more to one side or other of the abdomen may indicate the presence of a pelvic inflammatory condition, and his assessment should take this into account.

However, to return to our more detailed approach, dysmenorrhoea can mainly be distinguished as of two types – those due to an excess (Shi) condition – Liver – and those due to a deficiency (Xu) – Kidney.

Those due to a Shi condition can again be divided into three types:
  (a) Stagnation or Retardation of Qi
  (b) Stagnation of Blood
  (c) Stagnation due to Cold

**(a) Stagnation of Qi**
This is a condition frequently brought about by emotional disturbances, especially grief, worry and depression. This will block the Qi energy and thus cause the pain, which occurs *before* the onset of the menses. The patient will often feel more 'bloated' than painful, with a general feeling of heaviness in the chest and a strong feeling of distention in the lower abdomen. (Stagnation of Qi is marked more by distention than pain, stagnation of blood by pain rather than distention.). The breasts may be swollen and painful, and there will be increased irritability and a feeling of frustration and general pre-menstrual tension.

Because it is a Shi condition the patient will dislike pressure; because of the obstruction the flow, once it starts, will tend to be irregular but because of the absence of heat it will tend to be light. The blood will be darkish, sometimes with clots, and the pulse will be tense and wiry.

*Treatment*: This will be mainly to calm the Liver and to regulate the circulation of Qi and Blood:

> CV3 (Zhongji) to reduce excess in the Lower Jiao, to make the Qi run smoothly and to regulate the uterus.
> Sp8 (Diji) to regulate the flow of blood. Also has a special effect on the uterus.
> Li2 (Xingjian) circulates Qi and Blood in Liver and Gall Bladder.
> B132 (Ciliao) – 'experience' point.
> One could also consider CV6 (Qihai) to regulate the whole of the Qi and also to help the menses.

**(b) Stagnation of Blood**
This is characterized by the severity of the pain, which is severe, stabbing, and occurs mainly at the onset of and during the menses. It is concentrated in the lower abdomen but may radiate to the low back and the thighs and, because of the stagnation, is worse for pressure. The flow is not very heavy, but the blood is dark and clotted and the pain tends to subside once a large clot has been passed. In severe cases the Liver disharmony can produce vomiting of bile – in these cases there is often an associated imbalance on the Stomach.

The pulse will be deep and choppy, the tongue tending towards purplish with little fur.

*Treatment*: The main point to think of would naturally be CV3 (Zhongji) for regulating blood and Qi via the Lower Heater and because it has a specific connection with the uterus, and this point may be augmented with CV6 (Qihai) to affect the general Qi and to assist in removing the stagnation. Although it is a Shi condition and moxa would generally be contraindicated, we are dealing with a stagnant condition and I personally feel that the judicious use of heat on these two points is more efficacious than needling – perhaps even extending to the use of a moxa-box over the whole area embracing CV3 (Zhongji), CV4 (Guanyuan) and CV6 (Qihai).

Other obvious points are Sp10 (Xuehai) to

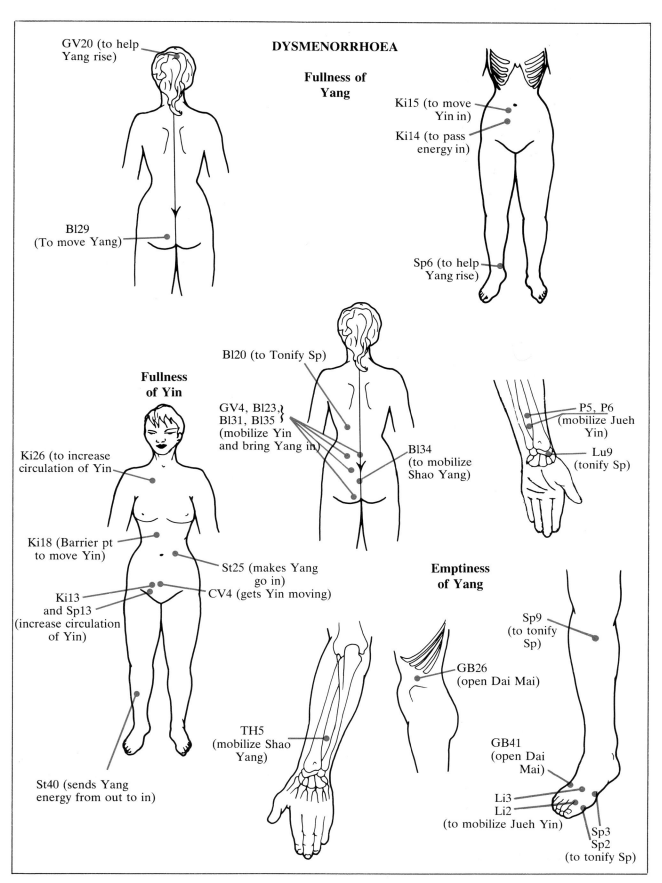

**DYSMENORRHOEA**

**Fullness of Yang**

GV20 (to help Yang rise)

Bl29 (To move Yang)

Ki15 (to move Yin in)

Ki14 (to pass energy in)

Sp6 (to help Yang rise)

**Fullness of Yin**

Bl20 (to Tonify Sp)

GV4, Bl23, Bl31, Bl35 (mobilize Yin and bring Yang in)

Bl34 (to mobilize Shao Yang)

P5, P6 (mobilize Jueh Yin)

Lu9 (tonify Sp)

Ki26 (to increase circulation of Yin

Ki18 (Barrier pt to move Yin)

St25 (makes Yang go in)

CV4 (gets Yin moving)

Ki13 and Sp13 (increase circulation of Yin)

**Emptiness of Yang**

Sp9 (to tonify Sp)

GB26 (open Dai Mai)

TH5 (mobilize Shao Yang)

St40 (sends Yang energy from out to in)

GB41 (open Dai Mai)

Li3
Li2 (to mobilize Jueh Yin)

Sp3
Sp2 (to tonify Sp)

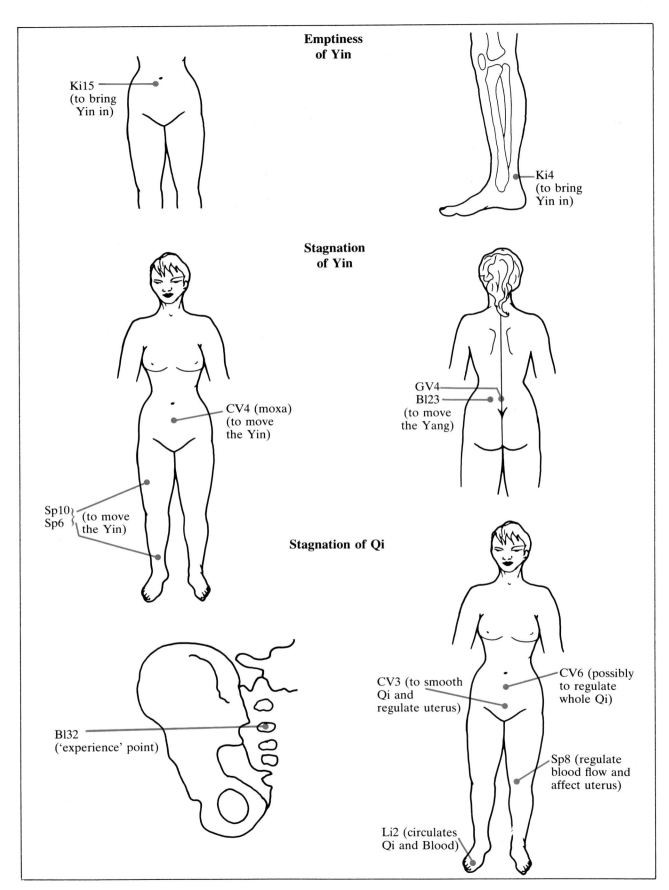

**Emptiness of Yin**

Ki15 (to bring Yin in)

Ki4 (to bring Yin in)

**Stagnation of Yin**

CV4 (moxa) (to move the Yin)

Sp10 } Sp6 } (to move the Yin)

GV4
Bl23 (to move the Yang)

**Stagnation of Qi**

Bl32 ('experience' point)

CV3 (to smooth Qi and regulate uterus)

CV6 (possibly to regulate whole Qi)

Sp8 (regulate blood flow and affect uterus)

Li2 (circulates Qi and Blood)

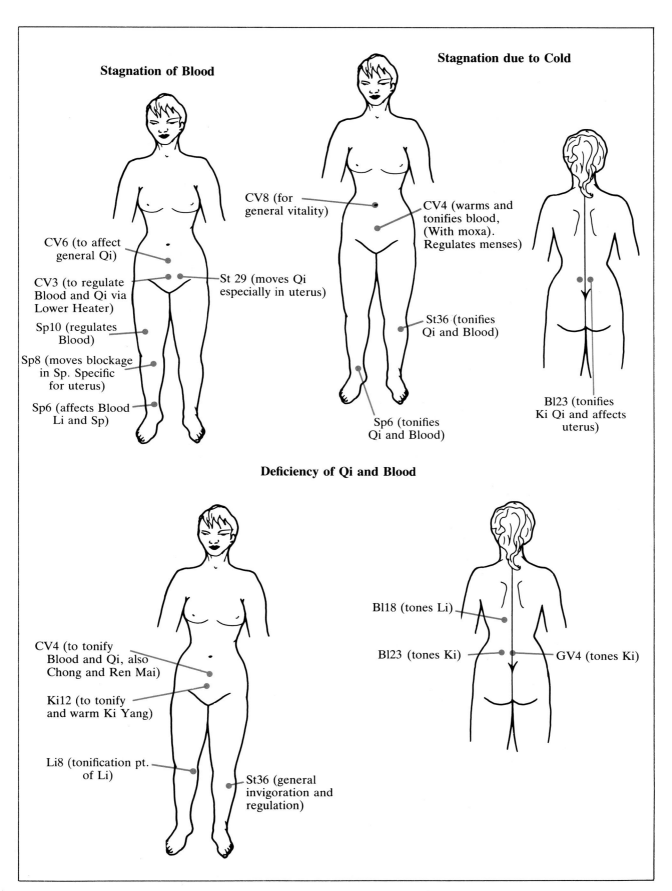

**Stagnation of Blood**

CV8 (for general vitality)

CV6 (to affect general Qi)

CV3 (to regulate Blood and Qi via Lower Heater)

St 29 (moves Qi especially in uterus)

Sp10 (regulates Blood)

Sp8 (moves blockage in Sp. Specific for uterus)

Sp6 (affects Blood Li and Sp)

**Stagnation due to Cold**

CV4 (warms and tonifies blood, (With moxa). Regulates menses)

St36 (tonifies Qi and Blood)

Sp6 (tonifies Qi and Blood)

Bl23 (tonifies Ki Qi and affects uterus)

**Deficiency of Qi and Blood**

CV4 (to tonify Blood and Qi, also Chong and Ren Mai)

Ki12 (to tonify and warm Ki Yang)

Li8 (tonification pt. of Li)

St36 (general invigoration and regulation)

Bl18 (tones Li)

Bl23 (tones Ki)

GV4 (tones Ki)

41

regulate the blood, St29 (Guilai) to move the Qi especially in the uterus, Sp6 (Sanyinjiao) for its specific effects on blood and on the liver and spleen, Sp4 (Gongsun) to open Chong Mai, and Sp8 (Diji). This latter, as the Xi-Cleft point of Spleen, is usually thought of where there is an acute blockage of Qi in the Spleen meridian and it, too, has a specific effect on the uterus. All these points should be used in reduction, but it is essential to keep the Dai Qi moving by manipulation every five minutes or so, since the essential thing is to keep the energy flowing and thus to relieve the stagnation.

### (c) Stagnation due to Cold

Although generally classified as a 'Shi' condition because it is due to an excess of cold, this manifests certain of the Xu characteristics of being better for warmth and pressure, although the initial touch may be resisted. Its aetiology is usually given as being due to living or working in cold conditions, or taking too much cold food and drink.

The pain usually occurs either just before or at the beginning of the period, and the flow is usually scanty with a tendency to thin, darkish blood with occasional clots. In some circumstances, however, the flow may be abundant, and the blood will then be more watery and the pain lasting for the whole of the menstrual cycle, which may last longer than normally. The pain itself is not so severe as in the preceding conditions, but consists of a dull dragging ache over the whole lower abdomen radiating to the low back and legs, which feel tired and aching. The pulse is deep and tight, and the tongue may have a whitish fur.

*Treatment:* There is Cold present, so we must obviously overcome this by the use of warmth, combined where necessary with needling to love the Qi and blood.

CV4 (Guanyuan) is the first point to think of – many authorities advocate needling first and then using moxa afterwards, but I have personally found the use of a heated needle very effective.

CV8 (Shenque) will improve the general vitality and is important for regulating the Ren Mai – naturally to be used only with the special technique applicable to this point of moxa on salt.

Sp6 (Sanyinjiao) and St36 (Zusanli) will tonify the Qi and also the blood (needle and moxa).

Bl23 (Shenshu) will tonify the Kidney Qi and have an effect upon the uterus (moxa).

There is only one *Xu* condition, and that is a deficiency of both Qi and blood. It is more rare than the Shi conditions, and is basically a deficiency of Kidney and Liver energy brought about by general weakness, either following a long illness, too many pregnancies, or possibly too great a blood loss with the menses.

The pain is dull rather than severe, and occurs either towards the end or after the menses; it is better for warmth and pressure. The blood is scanty and pinkish, and the patient is listless and tired with a sallow complexion. There may be dizziness, tinnitus, chilliness, constipation and ache in the low back – all signs of Kidney deficiency. The pulse is deep, thready and weak, the tongue pale.

*Treatment* Moxa CV4 (Guanyuan) to tonify blood and Qi. Will also tonify Chong Mai, Ren Mai, and the Liver and Kidney channels.

Tonify Bl18 (Ganshu) and Bl23 (Shenshu) and moxa after, to stimulate Liver and Kidney.

Needle and moxa St36 (Zusanli), for its general invigorating and regulatory effect.

Tonify Li8 (Ququan), the tonification point of Liver.

Moxa GV4 (Mingmen) for the Kidneys.

Needle and moxa Ki12 (Dahe) to tonify and warm the Kidney Yang.

In all cases of dysmenorrhoea it is usually advisable to initiate treatment three to five days before the commencement of the menses and to repeat during the actual periods, but I find also that as all treatments are directed towards encouraging the movement of blood and Qi, treatment during the 'quiescent' time between menses may prove beneficial in procuring a long-lasting effect. It is usual to advise the patient to keep warm during the time of the periods, and to avoid eating cold or too many raw foods.

# IRREGULAR MENSES

By these we mean menses which occur with either an early or a late cycle, or which are truly irregular, i.e. sometimes early, sometimes late.

It is easy to see that we are dealing with a question of the movement of blood and energy in time: overactivity = acceleration = too frequent periods; underactivity = stagnation = delayed menses.

This condition is usually associated with disturbances of Chong Mai, Ren Mai and one or other of the three Zu Yin lines – Kidney, Liver and Spleen channels.

If the Kidney is deficient the functions of Chong Mai and Ren Mai are upset.

If the Liver is affected by heat the organ cannot store the blood.

If the Spleen is deficient, the Spleen cannot produce blood.

## Early cyclic bleeding

This is usually a sign of Heat in the blood, and has two main causes:

(a) Emotional:
  (i) Anxiety, which coagulates the Qi. Long stagnation of Qi changes it into Fire, which causes early bleeding, or
  (ii) Anger, which causes Heat in the Liver, which fails to store the blood.
(b) The acute invasion of some external 'hot' factor which causes blood Heat which accumulates in the womb to cause early menses.

Diagnosis rests naturally upon the early appearance of the menses, which may even be as often as twice in the month, whilst the blood flow will be profuse with bright red blood. (If stagnation occurs the blood will tend to be darker in colour and may even present with clots). The pulse will be rapid (over 90 per minute) and wiry (deeper and more slippery if there is stagnation present); the tongue red, with yellow fur if the heat is coagulated. The patient will be irritable, with a flushed complexion, thirsty, possibly constipated with a dry stool and yellow urine.

*Treatment:* CV4 (Guanyuan) and CV6 (Qihai). (CV4 is a reunion point of the three Zu Yin lines and Ren Mai; CV6 regulates the Yuan Qi).

SP6 (Sanyinjiao) – regulates the three leg Yin.

Li3 (Taichong) (or Li2 (Xingjian) – regulates Liver Fire.

Ki3 (Taixi) – benefits the Kidney water.

Sp10 (Xuehai) – to cool the blood.

## Late cyclic bleeding

This may be up to fourteen to fifteen days late and is the result of a deficient and Cold condition. The Cold stays and stagnates in the uterus causing a deficiency of Yang and exhaustion of blood, affecting Chong Mai and Ren Mai.

Typically there will be a small amount of thin, light-coloured blood, and the patient will feel weak, with a pallid complexion and a desire for

# IRREGULAR MENSES

## Early Cyclic Bleeding

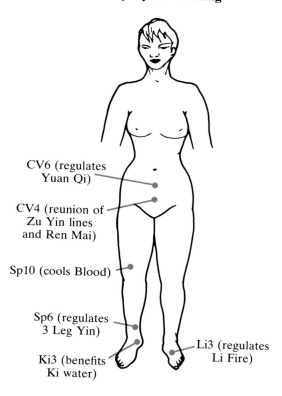

CV6 (regulates Yuan Qi)

CV4 (reunion of Zu Yin lines and Ren Mai)

Sp10 (cools Blood)

Sp6 (regulates 3 Leg Yin)

Ki3 (benefits Ki water)

Li3 (regulates Li Fire)

## Late Cyclic Bleeding

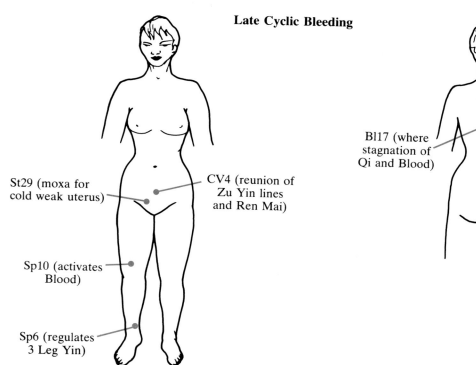

St29 (moxa for cold weak uterus)

CV4 (reunion of Zu Yin lines and Ren Mai)

Sp10 (activates Blood)

Sp6 (regulates 3 Leg Yin)

Bl17 (where stagnation of Qi and Blood)

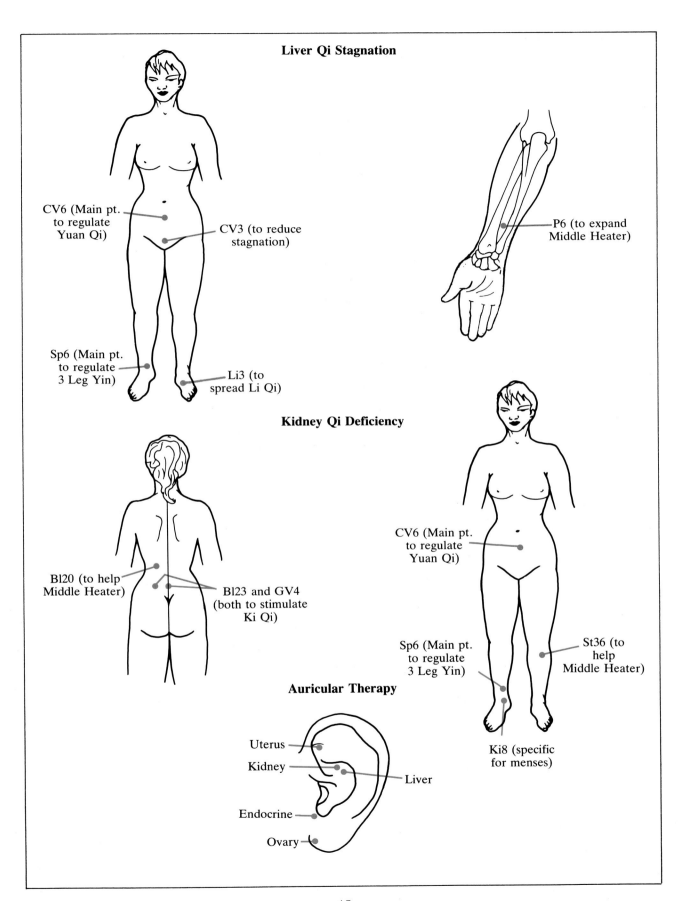

**Liver Qi Stagnation**

CV6 (Main pt. to regulate Yuan Qi)

CV3 (to reduce stagnation)

P6 (to expand Middle Heater)

Sp6 (Main pt. to regulate 3 Leg Yin)

Li3 (to spread Li Qi)

**Kidney Qi Deficiency**

Bl20 (to help Middle Heater)

Bl23 and GV4 (both to stimulate Ki Qi)

CV6 (Main pt. to regulate Yuan Qi)

Sp6 (Main pt. to regulate 3 Leg Yin)

St36 (to help Middle Heater)

Ki8 (specific for menses)

**Auricular Therapy**

Uterus

Kidney

Liver

Endocrine

Ovary

45

warmth. The pulse will be slow (under 60 per minute) and weak; the tongue will be pale with either no or thin white fur.

This typical picture, however, may be subject to variations, and acute invasion of Damp accompanying the Cold may obstruct the flow and cause the blood to become dark. The patient will frequently complain of accompanying pain in the low back. Similarly, a stagnation of Qi and blood will also result in dark blood, possibly with clots – in this case the tongue may become dark red and the pulse will become more wiry.

Treatment will, typically, consist of CV4 (Guanyuan) and Sp6 (Sanyinjiao), with the addition of Sp10 (Xuehai) to activate the blood and St29 (Guilai) for the cold and weak uterus. Needle for the stagnation and moxa for the deficiency. Where there is stagnation of Qi and blood one might consider the addition of Bl17 (Geshu).

## Irregular menses

Can be due to excess coitus, chronic haemorrhage, or a weakness of Stomach and Spleen affecting the Liver and Kidney Qi, which in turn will affect Chong Mai and Ren Mai. There is usually an over-use of Kidney Qi, although strong emotional disturbances can cause stagnation of Liver Qi. In this latter instance – stagnation of Liver Qi – there will be an irregular flow of dark, purplish blood, with pain in the lower abdomen before and/or after the menses. There may be congestion in the chest and belching. The tongue will be purplish or with purple spots, the pulse will be rough and wiry.

Where there is a Kidney Qi deficiency the blood will vary in quantity and will be pale. The patient will feel weak and tend to emaciation, with a withered yellowish complexion, whilst she may complain of backache and dizziness. The tongue will be pale, the pulse small and weak, possibly rough.

*Treatment:* Once more, the two basic points are CV6 (Qihai) and Sp6 (Sanyinjiao). Many authorities specify CV4 (Guanyuan), which has a more direct effect upon the menses, whilst CV6 will affect the Yuan Qi more generally. Further points are added according to the condition:

Liver Qi stagnation: P6 (Neiguan) to expand the Middle Heater.
Li3 (Taichong) to spread the Liver Qi.
CV3 (Zhongji) to reduce the stagnation.
Kidney Qi deficient: GV4 (Mingmen) to stimulate the Kidney Qi.
Bl23 (Shenshu) to stimulate the Kidney Qi.
Ki8 (Jiaoxin) for its specific effect upon the menses.

Bl20 (Pishu) and St36 (Zusanli) can be used to help the Middle Jiao to 'support the foundation of Qi and Blood'.
Useful auricular points could be Uterus, Endocrine, Ovary, Kidney, and Liver.

# ABNORMAL UTERINE BLEEDING

This condition is known in Chinese as Bung-Luo, Bung referring to an excessive flow outside the normal menstrual period, and Luo to an incessant constant dripping. In cases where there has been a sudden great loss of blood (as in an emergency situation) Bung may change into Luo, whilst under other circumstances Luo may change into Bung.

The recognized forms of abnormal uterine bleeding are:

Menorrhagia – an excessive bleeding with a normal length of cycle.

Metrorrhagia – irregular or continuous bleeding from the uterus at times other than the normal menstrual period.

Polymenorrhoea – frequent and often profuse menses with a shorter cycle.

Epimenorrhoea – intermittent bleeding – uterine bleeding apart from normal menstruation.

Oligomenorrhoea – scanty bleeding or longer cycle.

The various causes may be:

Lesions of the cervix: polypus, carcinoma, vascular erosion.

Lesions of the body of the uterus: endometritis, tuberculosis, fibroids, polypi, endometriosis, myohyperplasia, carcinoma, mixed mesodermal tumours, sarcoma.

Lesions of the ovary: oestrogen-secreting tumours, endometriosis, chronic infection.

Complications of pregnancy: abortion, ectopic pregnancy, hydatidiform mole, chorioncarcinoma.

Treatment with ovarian hormones may induce bleeding, especially in menopausal and post-menopausal women, whilst what is known as 'Breakthrough bleeding' may result from synthetic progestogens given for oral contraception or for the treatment of pelvic disorders.

A tendency to abnormal bleeding may be present in thrombocytopenic purpura and other blood dyscrasias; menorrhagia or irregular bleeding may result from hyper- or hypothyroidism. Psychosomatic causes, such as severe emotional shock, may also be responsible.

Metrorrhagia (an excessive flow of blood outside the normal menstrual period) can be due to either an excess of blood or to an excess of Yang energy (with therefore a relative deficiency of Yin at the pelvic level). Treatment based upon this concept would involve moving the plethora of blood and energy by the use of Sp13 (Fushe), Bl18 (Ganshu) and Bl19 (Danshu), whilst Li9 (Yinbao) will tonify the envelope of Yin. The Yin energy should be stimulated via CV3 (Zhongji), CV5 (Shimen), CV6 (Qihai) and Lu7 (Lieque), and the energy of Tai Yin and Jueh Yin via Sp6 (Sanyinjiao), Sp2 (Dadu) and Li2 (Xingjian).

From a TCM point of view, abnormal bleeding is due to inabilities of the Liver to store and of the Spleen to hold the blood, and to disruption of the functions of Chong Mai and Ren Mai in controlling the blood flow. The Kidney dominates the storage of blood, and it is therefore these channels and organs which are the targets for treatment.

Various factors may be responsible – excess coitus can damage the Kidney Qi and hence produce dysfunction of Chong Mai and Ren Mai. Anxiety can upset the Liver function, leading to stagnation of Qi and blood to produce heat. The 'evil heat' can stagnate the blood which will flow outside its usual time. Faulty diet or excessive worry can cause a deficiency in the Spleen Qi which will fail to control the blood and will thus give rise to dripping.

We thus see that there can be a number of causative factors, each of which can produce a specific imbalance which, as it develops, will affect the other channels and pathways and either the excess (Shi) of Yang or the deficiency (Xu) of Yin will preponderate.

## The Shi type

This will be predominantly an excess of Heat in the Liver, and will manifest as a heavy flow of deep red blood with a foetid odour. This will be accompanied by abdominal pain worse for pressure, a dry mouth, and possibly constipation, whilst the Liver involvement can affect the Heart and give rise to irritability. The pulse will be big and rapid, the tongue red with a yellowish coating.

If the blood tends to stagnate then there will be a concomitant formation of clots, and the abdominal pain will lessen after they have been passed. Although the tongue proper will be deep red, there will be little coating.

*Treatment:* In the Shi type, heat predominates, so moxa is contra-indicated and reducing techniques are used.

The principal points are:
> CV4 (Guanyuan) to regulate Chong Mai and Ren Mai.
>
> Sp6 (Sanyinjiao) to regulate the Spleen, the Zu Yin lines, and the blood.
>
> Sp1 (Yinbai) – the 'welling-point' of Spleen, to strengthen its Qi, also an 'experience' point for uterine bleeding.

whilst we add:
> Sp10 (Xuehai) to clear Heat in the blood.

> Ki5 (Shuiquan) to disperse Heat in the blood.
>
> Bl120 (Pishu) – the Back-Shu point of Spleen.
>
> Li1 (Dadun) to clear Heat in the Liver and blood,

and possibly stimulate St36 (Zusanli) to reinforce the basic Qi.

## The Xu type

This consists basically of either Spleen Qi Xu or Kidney Qi Xu, the latter being of either Kidney Yang or Kidney Yin. Both Spleen Qi Xu and Kidney Yang Xu can produce either a profuse or a 'Luo' – a constant dripping – flow of blood, which is light red in colour.

Mainly, however, the Qi Xu type is characterized by a long, steady dripping of dark red blood, the patient having a pale face and no appetite or energy and feeling very weak. The pulse will be slow and tiny and the tongue pale with a slippery coat.

The Yin Xu is characterized by a lightish, scarlet blood, dizziness, tinnitus (Yin deficiency), palpitations, insomnia, and flushes in the afternoons. The pulse is deep and weak and the tongue red with no fur.

There is a fourth, very rare, Yin condition, known as the 'prostration' type. This will usually constitute a hospital emergency and is brought on by massive haemorrhage. The patient is pale and in shock, with a cold sweat and rapid breathing. The legs are cold and the pulse is too weak to find.

*Treatment:* This utilizes the same three basic points as used in the Shi type – CV4 (Guanyuan), Sp6 (Sanyinjiao) and Sp1 (Yinbai), but now we must stimulate and/or moxa.

For the Qi Xu type we add Bl20 (Pishu) and St36 (Zusanli) to reinforce the basic Qi.

For the Yin Xu type we add P6 (Neiguan) and Ki3 (Taixi) to reinforce the basic Yin (needle only).

For the prostration type we add GV20 (Baihui) and CV6 (Qihai), moxa, to help the Yuan Qi.

If considering auricular therapy, use Uterus, Endocrine, and Dermis (Sub-Cortex). Retain the needles in situ for 1 to 2 hours, with intermittent stimulation.

# ABNORMAL UTERINE BLEEDING

### Shi Type

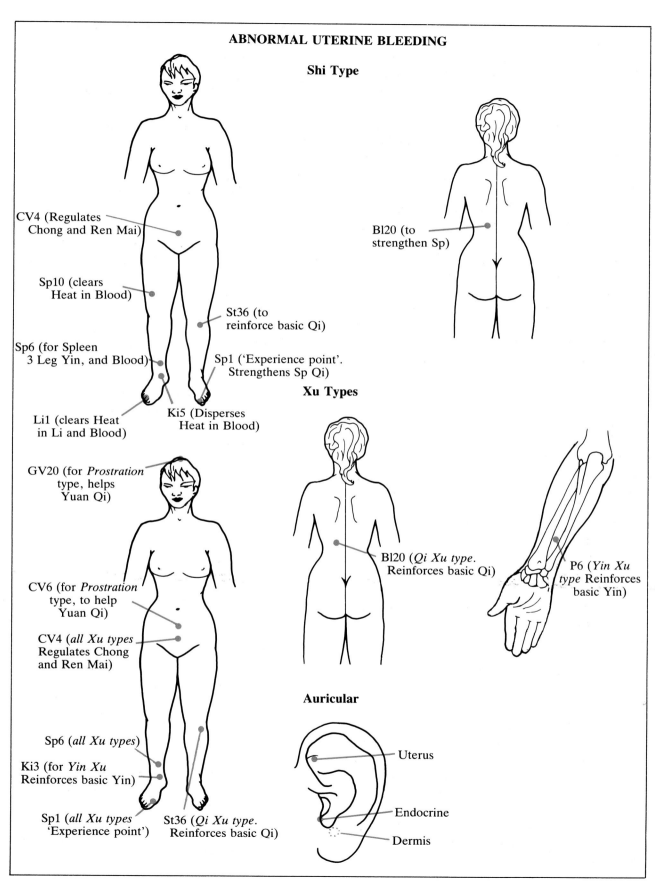

CV4 (Regulates Chong and Ren Mai)

Sp10 (clears Heat in Blood)

St36 (to reinforce basic Qi)

Sp6 (for Spleen 3 Leg Yin, and Blood)

Sp1 ('Experience point'. Strengthens Sp Qi)

Li1 (clears Heat in Li and Blood)

Ki5 (Disperses Heat in Blood)

Bl20 (to strengthen Sp)

### Xu Types

GV20 (for *Prostration* type, helps Yuan Qi)

CV6 (for *Prostration* type, to help Yuan Qi)

CV4 (*all Xu types* Regulates Chong and Ren Mai)

Sp6 (*all Xu types*)

Ki3 (for *Yin Xu* Reinforces basic Yin)

Sp1 (*all Xu types* 'Experience point')

St36 (*Qi Xu type*. Reinforces basic Qi)

Bl20 (*Qi Xu type*. Reinforces basic Qi)

P6 (*Yin Xu type* Reinforces basic Yin)

### Auricular

Uterus

Endocrine

Dermis

49

# LEUCORRHOEA

It is quite normal for there to be a slight vaginal discharge, there being a small watery one from the uterine lining, a whitish one from the cervical glands, and a white acid secretion from the vagina, the glands of Bartholin and the vulva. This is inoffensive, and is increased just before the menstrual period, especially if there is pelvic congestion due to constipation. It is only when they are excessive in amount that they are termed leucorrhoea, and they may then become offensive, purulent or blood-stained.

From a Western viewpoint, the most looked-for cause is an infective agent, notably Trichomona vaginalis or some bacillary infection. Other causes may be gonorrhoeal cervicitis, endometritis or salpingitis. A bloodstained discharge may result from fibroid polypi, whilst cancer of the uterus will often first demonstrate as a thin, watery, bloodstained discharge which later becomes thick, purulent and offensive. Any growth such as a tumour which can cause pelvic congestion can also cause leucorrhoea, so it is incumbent upon the practitioner to rule out any cause which will not be amenable to acupuncture before considering treatment. Excessive oestrogen may also instigate leucorrhoea.

From the standpoint of TCM, there are three fundamental causes. The first one is local, and embraces either pathology as considered in the previous paragraph or a disturbance in meridial energy, particularly the Liver with Damp-Cold or Damp-Heat forming mucus, or a deficiency of Kidney or Spleen energy.

The second cause is dysfunction of the Irregular Vessels – notably Chong Mai, Ren Mai and Dai Mai. The Yinqiao may also be involved.

The third cause is a disturbance in the movement of energy generally. This latter may manifest as either:

(a) Generalized Fullness of Yin
(b) Local Fullness of Yin (from stagnation)
(c) Emptiness of Yang
(d) Stagnation of Yang

### (a) Generalized Fullness of Yin
Better for Heat, worse for pressure and Cold; more to the right than to the left.
Use CV4 (Guanyuan), CV6 (Qihai), Sp6 (Sanyinjiao), GB26 (Daimai) and Ki18 (Shiguan).

### (b) Local Fullness of Yin, causing stagnation
Better for Heat and movement, worse for Cold and rest.
Use Sp13 (Fushe) to move the trunk Yin.
B133 (Zhongliao) or B134 (Xialiao) – Liao points of GB and Bl.
Ki6 (Zhaohai) and Ki8 (Jiaoxin) to move the Yingiao.

## (c) Emptiness of Yang

Better for Heat and pressure, worse for Cold and movement. General coldness and weakness, lack of appetite, watery stools, polyuria. Slow and Deep pulse, pale tongue with a thin greyish coating.

Use St29 (Guilai) and St25 (Tianshu) to make the Yang go in and down.

GV3 (Yaoyangguan) to make the Yang come down.

Bl32 (Ciliao) – Liao point.

## (d) Stagnation of Yang

Better for Heat and movement.

Use Bl27 (Xiaochangshu), which works on Dai Mai and the Shao Yang to move the Yang.

Bl56 (Chengjin), Bl57 (Chengshan) and Bl58 (Feiyang), with massage before needling, to move blocked energy in the upper part of the body.

And either GB41 (Linqi) for Dai Mai *or* Bl62 (Shenmai) for the Yangqiao according to the case.

## Disturbance of the Irregular Vessels

As stated previously, the Irregular Vessels most likely to be involved are Chong Mai, Ren Mai and Dai Mai. Chong Mai, as the 'Sea of Blood', plays an integral role in governing the flow of blood and Qi; Ren Mai governs the energy of the Yin meridians and will thus affect the energy of the kidney and liver organs; Dai Mai, as the girdle vessel, will govern free movement of energy between the upper and the lower parts of the body, and is particularly important where there is a stagnation of Yang in the pelvic basin – dysfunction of this vessel will often produce the oft-cited symptom of 'sensation of sitting in water', but it can also cause pain in the umbilical area radiating to the lumbar area or to the internal thigh.

The Yinqiao is occasionally involved in that it is responsible for the transport of Jing energy. Dysfunction of this vessel may manifest with concomitant pain and redness in the eyes, emanating from the internal canthus, also a contraction of the internal thighs with relaxation of the external and radiating pains in the lower abdomen.

Treatment of the Yinqiao would involve points Ki6 (Zhaohai) and Ki8 (Jiaoxin), and if there are symptoms of Yin in the interior, stimulation of St36 (Zusanli).

## Local causes

In considering these, we must not forget the state of the vaginal mucosa. A depletion of energy from either the kidney or the spleen may cause an issue to the exterior, and possible points to help this could be Sp3 (Taibai) and Sp4 (Gongsun) to affect the Tai Yin, and Li5 (Ligou), which commands the mucosa itself. If Damp-Heat is present, add Sp16 (Fuai), if Damp-Cold, add Sp19 (Xiongxiang).

The chief and simplest differentiation of the cause is whether there is (a) White, or (b) Yellowish, discharge.

## (a) White (Bai Dai)

This is due to a deficiency of Qi and the presence of Damp. The discharge is white, thin and watery, and may be due to:

(i) Weakness of Kidney Yang, when the discharge is described as being 'like the white of an egg', slow, and slightly abundant. There will be soft stools and copious and clear urine, general weakness, and possibly a severe backache. The tongue is pale and white, the pulse deep and fine.

(ii) Weakness of Kidney Yin. Although placed under the heading of a 'white' discharge, the discharge here may be reddish, because tinged with blood which circulates in a disorderly manner due to the false-fire which accumulates. There will be general weakness, possibly vertigo and/or tinnitus, or palpitations. The tongue will be clear and red, the pulse fine and rapid.

(iii) Weakness in the Spleen, usually due to faulty eating and tiredness. Lack of pure energy to the Middle Heater interferes with the transformation of blood which, instead of ascending to the heart, descends to form damp fluids which manifest as leucorrhoea. The discharge is thin, watery and odourless (like a nasal discharge). The patient has weak, cold limbs with a tendency to oedema pedum, soft stools, a clear and copious urine. The tongue is pale and flabby, the pulse weak and retarded.

(iv) Damp-Phlegm. An accumulation of Yin dampness due to lack of Spleen energy causes a general weakness in the circulation of Yang through the whole body. The discharges are slimy and abundant, the patient usually obese with abdominal distention, with a heavy head, tinnitus, an insipid taste in the mouth, nausea, little appetite, dyspnoea, and is catarrhal. The tongue is pale and damp and the pulse slippery.

## (b) Yellow (Huang Dai)

Due to a downwards infusion of Damp-Heat. Dysfunction of Ren Mai and Dai Mai allow a downward flow of perverse humidity to accumulate in the pelvic basin, causing leucorrhoea.

The discharge is abundant, deep yellow and probably pinkish, thick and viscous, with a foetid odour. There is restlessness and irritability, possibly palpitations, a dry mouth with scanty saliva, and what can only be described as 'abnormal' stools – soft, but constipated, and an 'unsatisfactory' urging. The urine is red, sometimes frequent and painful, with urethritis. The tongue is yellow and moist, the pulse superficial and rapid.

*Treatment:* The treatment of all cases is based upon a group of specific points to be used in all instances, with subsidiary ones to be added according to the cause.

The basic points are: GB26 (Daimai) and GB41 (Linqi) to regulate Dai Mai.

> Sp6 (Sanyinjiao) to regulate the Zuyin lines and eliminate damp.
> CV6 (Qihai) to strengthen the Qi via Ren Mai and Chong Mai, and to help retain the fluids.
> St29 (Guilai) may be considered as a specific local point.

The subsidiary points are:
(i) Weakness of Kidney Yang – Bl23 (Shenshu), CV6 (Qihai), Ki2 (Rangu), GV4 (Mingmen). St36 (Zusanli) to strengthen Qi and blood.
(ii) Weakness of Kidney Yin – Ki3 (Taixi), Ki7 (Fuliu), Ki10 (Yingu), Bl32 (Ciliao) ('experience' point) and CV4 (Guanyuan)
(iii) Weakness in Spleen – Bl20 (Pishu), St36 (Zusanli), CV4 (Guanyuan)
(iv) Damp-Phlegm – Bl20 (Pishu), St36 (Zusanli), Sp2 (Dadu), St40 (Fenglong)

to transform mucus.
(v) Damp-Heat (Huang Dai) – Sp9 (Yinlingquan) strengthens Spleen
Li2 (Xingjian) eliminates Liver fire
CV3 (Zhongji) and Li5 (Ligou) reduce Liver fire

In auricular therapy the same points are utilized in all cases: Uterus, Ovary, Internal secretion, and Shenmen.

Apart from the differentiation into white and yellow discharges, there is a third, less usual, one characterized by a reddish discharge (Chi Dai) sometimes tinged with white. If it is predominately red, care must be taken to distinguish it from mid-cycle bleeding or, if very profuse, from a uterine haemorrhage.

Traditionally there are two basic causes:

(a) Damp Heat, or
(b) Deficiency of blood.

*(a) Damp Heat,* In many respects this is extremely similar to the Damp-Heat yellow discharge (Huang Dai), but in this instance the damp-heat is caused by a weakness of Spleen function associated with Liver disturbance. It presents with a repulsive-smelling continuous reddish, purulent discharge. As with all heat conditions, there will be thirst, concentrated urine, and possibly a bitter taste in the mouth. The tongue is red with a thickish yellow coating, the pulse slippery and rapid.

Treatment would consist of moving the damp and supporting the functions of Liver, Spleen and Dai Mai: Sp6 (Sanyinjiao), Sp9 (Yinlingquan), Li2 (Xingjian), CV6 (Qihai) and GB26 (Daimai) for Dai Mai. We could possibly augment also with the key point for Dai Mai, GB41 (Linqi).

*(b) Deficiency of blood.* This is a Shi condition brought about by an excess of Heart and Liver Fire 'drying' the blood. The discharge will be scanty, but still with a repulsive odour. There will be thirst, possibly constipation with dry faeces, precordial pain and heartburn. Although there is a deficiency of blood the tongue may tend to be darkish from the Heart Fire, but could also appear pale and dry. The pulse is usually thready and rapid.

The treatment is to reduce the heart and

liver fire and to open Dai Mai, also to stimulate the Spleen and Kidney.

Stimulate Sp6 (Sanyinjiao), CV4 (Guanyuan), CV6 (Qihai), GB26 (Daimai), with Bl17 (Geshu), Bl20 (Pishu) and Bl23 (Shenshu).

Reduce Li2 (Xingjian) and Ht8 (Shaofu).

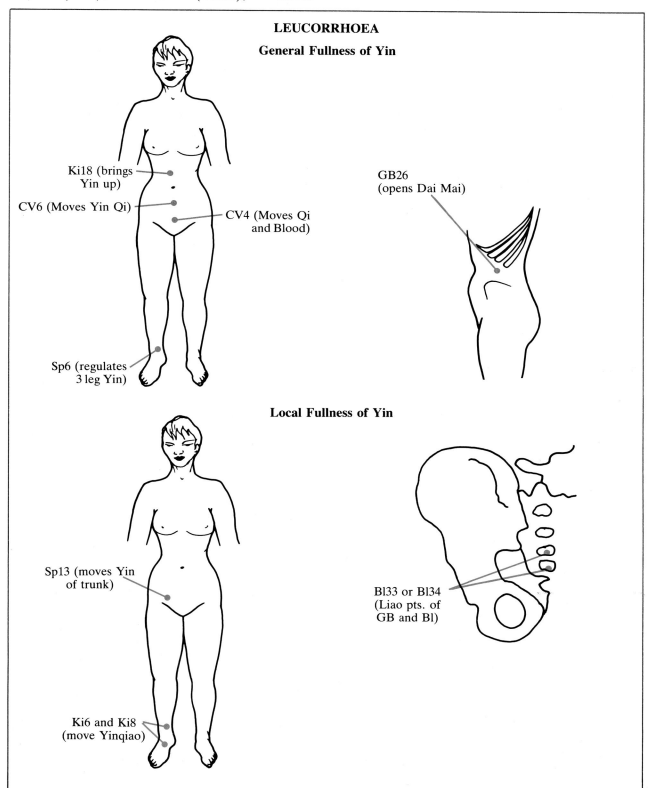

**LEUCORRHOEA**

**General Fullness of Yin**

Ki18 (brings Yin up)

CV6 (Moves Yin Qi)

CV4 (Moves Qi and Blood)

GB26 (opens Dai Mai)

Sp6 (regulates 3 leg Yin)

**Local Fullness of Yin**

Sp13 (moves Yin of trunk)

Bl33 or Bl34 (Liao pts. of GB and Bl)

Ki6 and Ki8 (move Yinqiao)

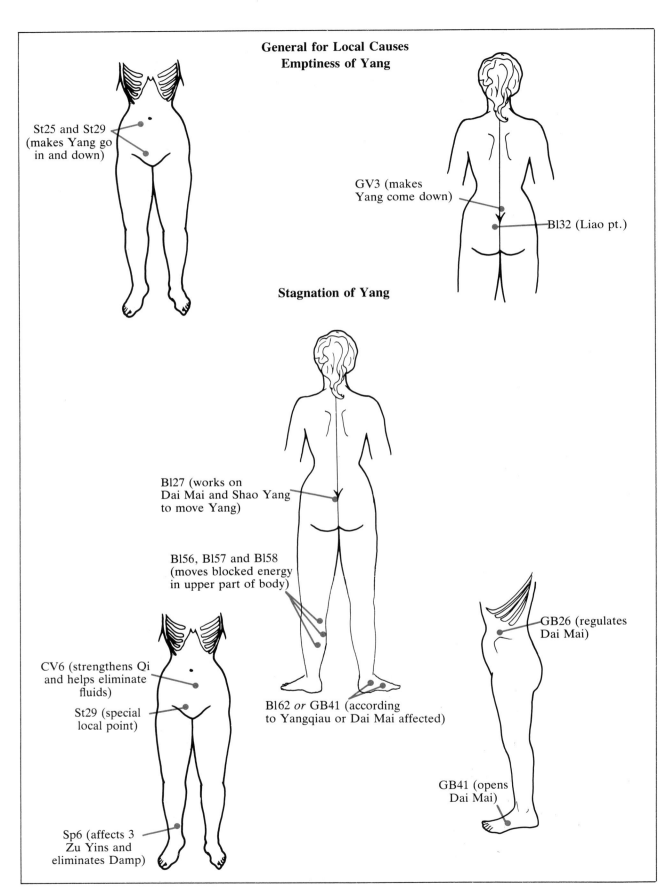

**General for Local Causes**
**Emptiness of Yang**

St25 and St29
(makes Yang go
in and down)

GV3 (makes
Yang come down)

Bl32 (Liao pt.)

**Stagnation of Yang**

Bl27 (works on
Dai Mai and Shao Yang
to move Yang)

Bl56, Bl57 and Bl58
(moves blocked energy
in upper part of body)

GB26 (regulates
Dai Mai)

CV6 (strengthens Qi
and helps eliminate
fluids)

St29 (special
local point)

Bl62 *or* GB41 (according
to Yangqiau or Dai Mai affected)

GB41 (opens
Dai Mai)

Sp6 (affects 3
Zu Yins and
eliminates Damp)

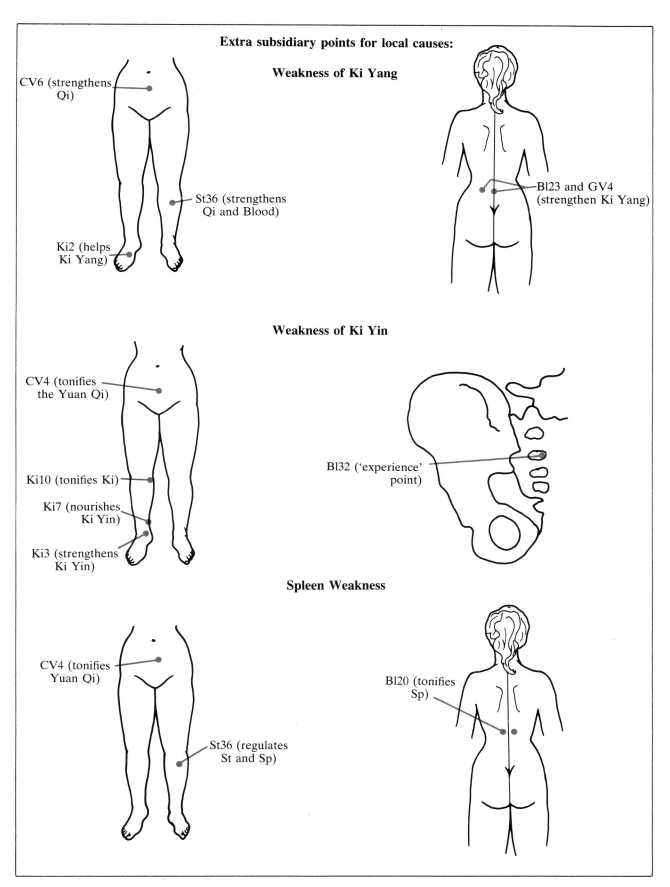

**Extra subsidiary points for local causes:**

**Weakness of Ki Yang**

CV6 (strengthens Qi)

St36 (strengthens Qi and Blood)

Ki2 (helps Ki Yang)

Bl23 and GV4 (strengthen Ki Yang)

**Weakness of Ki Yin**

CV4 (tonifies the Yuan Qi)

Ki10 (tonifies Ki)

Ki7 (nourishes Ki Yin)

Ki3 (strengthens Ki Yin)

Bl32 ('experience' point)

**Spleen Weakness**

CV4 (tonifies Yuan Qi)

St36 (regulates St and Sp)

Bl20 (tonifies Sp)

**Damp-Phlegm**

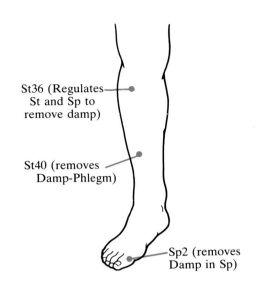

St36 (Regulates St and Sp to remove damp)

St40 (removes Damp-Phlegm)

Sp2 (removes Damp in Sp)

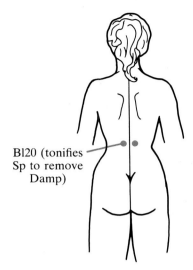

Bl20 (tonifies Sp to remove Damp)

**Damp-Heat**

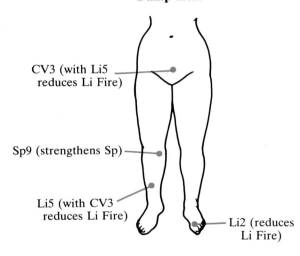

CV3 (with Li5 reduces Li Fire)

Sp9 (strengthens Sp)

Li5 (with CV3 reduces Li Fire)

Li2 (reduces Li Fire)

**Auricular Therapy**

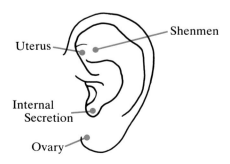

Uterus

Shenmen

Internal Secretion

Ovary

56

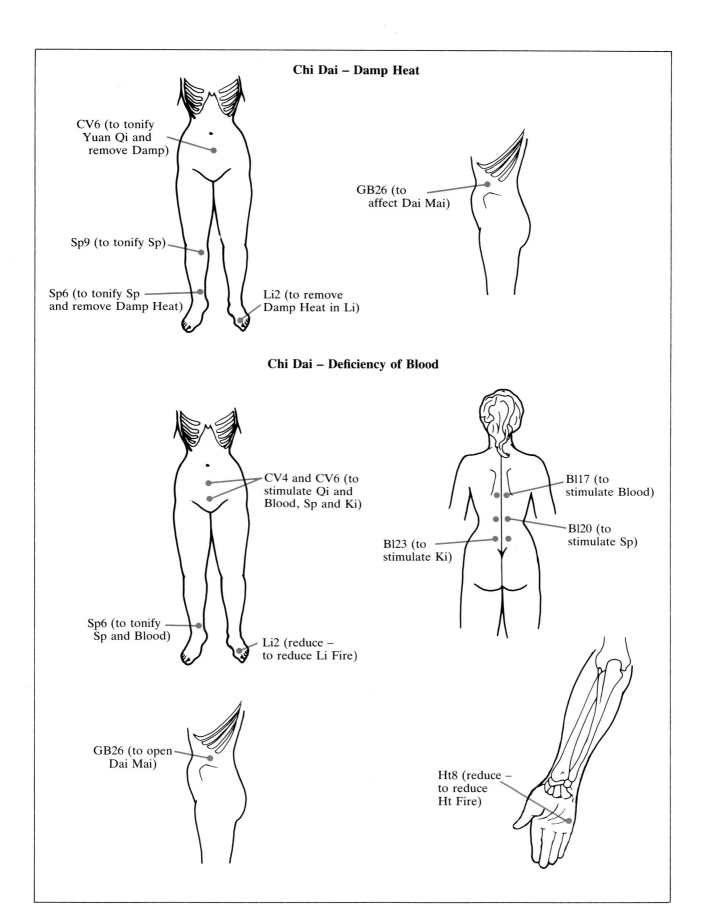

**Chi Dai – Damp Heat**

CV6 (to tonify Yuan Qi and remove Damp)

GB26 (to affect Dai Mai)

Sp9 (to tonify Sp)

Sp6 (to tonify Sp and remove Damp Heat)

Li2 (to remove Damp Heat in Li)

**Chi Dai – Deficiency of Blood**

CV4 and CV6 (to stimulate Qi and Blood, Sp and Ki)

Bl17 (to stimulate Blood)

Bl20 (to stimulate Sp)

Bl23 (to stimulate Ki)

Sp6 (to tonify Sp and Blood)

Li2 (reduce – to reduce Li Fire)

GB26 (to open Dai Mai)

Ht8 (reduce – to reduce Ht Fire)

# ENDOMETRIOSIS

Endometriosis is a condition wherein the tissues of the normal endometrial lining of the uterus are found outside the uterus (although there is the condition of internal endometriosis, or uterine adenomyosis, where the endometrium is found in the muscular wall of the uterus).

How the endometrial tissues come to be outside the uterus is not yet fully established, but there are three main theories:

(a) The embolic theory, whereby endometrial emboli may travel outside the uterus via the pelvic veins and lymphatics.
(b) The implantation theory, which claims that a retrograde menstruation may carry endometrial cells through the Fallopian tubes into the ovaries and other adjacent sites. (This theory fails to explain implantation into such remote sites as the pleura, kidneys, diaphragm or even the limbs, as has occasionally – although very rarely – been reported.)
(c) The serosal heteroplasia theory, based upon the fact that the germinal epithelial of the ovary and the pelvic peritoneum all arise from the coelonic tissue forming the Müllerian ducts and hence the uterus, tubes and upper part of the vagina, which presupposes that extra-uterine tissue could change into uterine type epithelium.

It has also been suggested that endometrial tissue might conceivably be transferred during surgery, but the commonest viewpoint would almost certainly be that of the implantation or retrograde flow theory.

Endometrial deposits can vary from the extremely small to the large 'chocolate cyst'. In this latter condition the tissue undergoes the usual endometrial bleeding but, because the blood cannot escape, a large cyst is formed. Perforation of this can lead to adhesions in the surrounding tissues leading, in advanced cases, to the so-called 'frozen pelvis'.

With the rare exceptions mentioned earlier, the usual sites are in the tissues of the pelvic basin, the commonest being in the ovaries. Other sites can include the pelvic peritoneum, the external uterus, the Fallopian tubes, the pouch of Douglas, the utero-sacral ligaments (possibly involving the recto-vaginal septum and posterior vaginal fornix), the round ligaments, the bowel (both large and small intestines), the bladder and uterus and the abdominal wall.

The commonest clinical picture is of fixed retroversion of the uterus, and uterine fibroids are often found in association with endometriosis.

The symptoms vary enormously, depending upon the sites and chronicity of the condition.

Pain may be that of a congestive type dysmenorrhoea, beginning a few days before the menses to be relieved once the flow is established, and felt in the pelvis and low back, or it may be the so-called 'Mittelschmertz' or pain at ovulation. The third type of pain is dyspareunia, felt deep in the pelvis and due to pressure on the ovaries and recto-vaginal septum.

Pain with bowel movements and on intercourse is common, whilst sterility is a frequent cause of complaint. In this latter case, indeed, the patient may not complain of pain at all, and come for consultation purely because of the failure to conceive – the tubes are usually patent, but the ovaries will be found to be palpably enlarged.

Menorrhagia is common, with short cycles and prolonged bleeding. This could possibly be due to the presence of fibroids, whilst the patient will frequently complain of general tiredness especially at the time of the periods, when there may even be a slight fever (possibly associated with fresh bleeding into the lesions).

Endometriosis of the bladder may cause haematuria at the time of menstruation.

Because endometriosis is non-malignant, and tends to regress at the time of the menopause, Western treatment is usually conservative, surgery being resorted to only in severe cases, when the endometrial tissue alone is removed and at least some ovarian tissue is left if at all possible.

It has been found that the endometrial deposits tend to regress during the second half of pregnancy and disappear after delivery, and it therefore seemed logical to use hormone administration to produce a state of pseudo-pregnancy and amenorrhoea – the usual choice is a progestational steroid Primolut-N (Norethisterone). Occasionally breakthrough bleeding may occur, and this is treated with either Ethinyl Oestrodiol or Danazol. This latter suppresses the hypothalaso-pituitary axis.

As a rough rule of thumb, pain before a period is due to stagnation of Qi, pain during a period is due to stagnation of blood, pain after is due to deficient blood and Qi. In endometriosis, as we have seen, the pain is either before (sometimes persisting through) the period, or else at ovulation. The former case will point to stagnation of either Qi or blood or both, and treatment must necesarily be directed accordingly.

Stagnation of Qi will produce distention in breasts and abdomen, stagnation of blood a severe pain at the onset of and during the menses; stagnation of Qi a tense and wiry pulse, stagnation of blood a deep and choppy one. In endometriosis, as distinct from dysmenorrhoea, it is the stagnation of the blood which is the predominant factor, but as 'the Qi moves the blood' we must concentrate on moving this also. The points chosen would be the usual ones for this sort of condition:

CV4 (Guanyuan) to move the blood
CV6 (Qihai) to move the Qi
Li3 (Taichong) to circulate Qi and blood
Sp8 (Diji) to regulate the flow of blood
St29 (Guilai) to move the Qi in the area
Sp6 (Sanyinjiao) to move the blood in the Zu Yin lines.

If the 'stagnation' proceeds for too long a time an accumulation of heat may occur, giving a feverish-type picture with a general restlessness and thirst and a yellow coating to the tongue. The abdominal pain will be better for the application of cold.

Points to move the blood and reduce the heat will be selected:

Sp10 (Xuehai) harmonizes and cools the blood
Li2 (Xingjian) removes heat in the Liver
St29 (Guilai) as a local point with its specific action on blood and Qi
TH6 )Zhigou) to disperse stuck blood
St25 (Tianshu) to regulate Qi and generally reduce 'stuckness' in the lower abdomen.

As with the condition of dysmenorrhoea known as 'Stagnation due to Cold', so endometriosis can present with a picture of stagnation of blood due to cold, with a dull nagging ache in the lower abdomen, better for warmth, and a flow of darkish blood with occasional clots. The pulse and tongue will have a similar picture to the stagnation due to cold – deep tight pulse and a whitish furred tongue.

Treatment will be directed to the same ends – move the blood and warm the cold, with points such as CV4 (Guanyuan), Sp6 (Sanyinjiao), Sp2 (Dadu) – Fire point of Spleen warms the blood – St30 (Qichong) (to remove blockage in Chong Mai), and Sp12 (Chongmen) (Barrier point to remove Yin in the pelvic basin).

# ENDOMETRIOSIS

## Stagnation of Blood

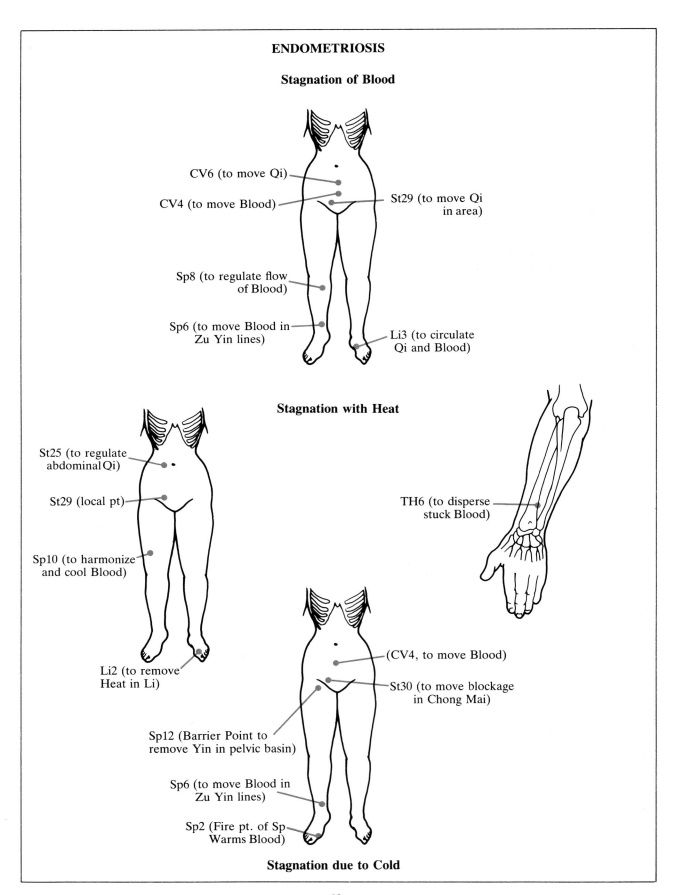

CV6 (to move Qi)

CV4 (to move Blood)

St29 (to move Qi in area)

Sp8 (to regulate flow of Blood)

Sp6 (to move Blood in Zu Yin lines)

Li3 (to circulate Qi and Blood)

## Stagnation with Heat

St25 (to regulate abdominal Qi)

St29 (local pt)

Sp10 (to harmonize and cool Blood)

TH6 (to disperse stuck Blood)

Li2 (to remove Heat in Li)

(CV4, to move Blood)

St30 (to move blockage in Chong Mai)

Sp12 (Barrier Point to remove Yin in pelvic basin)

Sp6 (to move Blood in Zu Yin lines)

Sp2 (Fire pt. of Sp Warms Blood)

## Stagnation due to Cold

# PRE-MENSTRUAL TENSION

This can be an extremely depressing condition. The commonest cause is depression of Liver Qi, which leads to a condition of stagnation giving rise to the depression. The depression of Qi can lead to an uprising of Liver Fire which will cause irritability and possibly swelling and pain in the breasts.

Treatment will obviously be directed towards promoting a smooth flowing of the Qi, the most usual points being Bl18 (Ganshu) and Bl19 (Danshu) as the Back-Shu points of the Liver and Gall Bladder, Li3 (Taichong) as the source point, Li14 (Qimen) the Front-Mu point, with Sp6 (Sanyinjiao) to move the Qi in the Zu Yin lines generally. Ki3 (Taixi) and P7 (Daling) are helpful for the pain in the breasts, whilst the use of GB41 (Linqi) can be considered if we feel we need to open Dai Mai.

When there is great tiredness and lassitude, possible with oedema of the legs, the cause is usually Spleen and Kidney Xu. Treatment would need to strengthen the spleen and the kidney, and traditionally consists of moxa to Bl20 (Pishu), Bl23 (Shenshu), and GV4 (Mingmen), and needle and moxa to CV4 (Guanyuan) and St36 (Zusanli). The reason for the selection of these points is obvious.

Dizziness, poor sleep, and possible palpitations, point to Spleen and Heart Xu, and treatment would utilize Bl15 (Xinshu) and Bl20 (Pishu) to tonify heart and spleen, Ht7 (Shenmen) for palpitations, Yintang (non-meridial point) if excessive dreaming, and CV6 (Qihai), St36 (Zusanli) and Sp6 (Sanyinjiao) to regulate the Qi.

The often-associated symptom of pain in the breasts is from the same root cause, depression of Liver Qi (collaterals of the Liver meridian supply the nipples). The prescription would include CV17 (Shanzhong) and St18 (Rugen) as local points, P6 (Neiguan) to affect the area, Li3 (Taichong), and St34 (Liangqui) (This point has a specific effect upon the breasts generally).

Occasionally, if the pain in the breasts is of an itching nature, possibly accompanied by a slight discharge, it may be due to stagnation of Liver and Stomach Fire. In this case the underlying condition could register on the pulse and tongue, giving a red tongue with a dry yellow coating and a rapid and wiry pulse. We could use similar points to those above, but include Li2 (Xingjian) instead of Li3 (Taichong).

In all cases of pre-menstrual tension the use of Ki5 (Shuiquan) can be considered, as this is an 'experience' point for this condition, whilst if it is desired to add points for general tension GV8 (Jinsue), GV12 (Shonzhu) and SI3 (Houxi) may prove of use, but it must be realized that these points will depress the Yang and as, predominately, pre-menstrual tension is a Xu condition, any reduction of Yang must be thought of carefully in its relationship to the whole energic balance.

# PRE-MENSTRUAL TENSION

## To promote smooth flowing of Qi

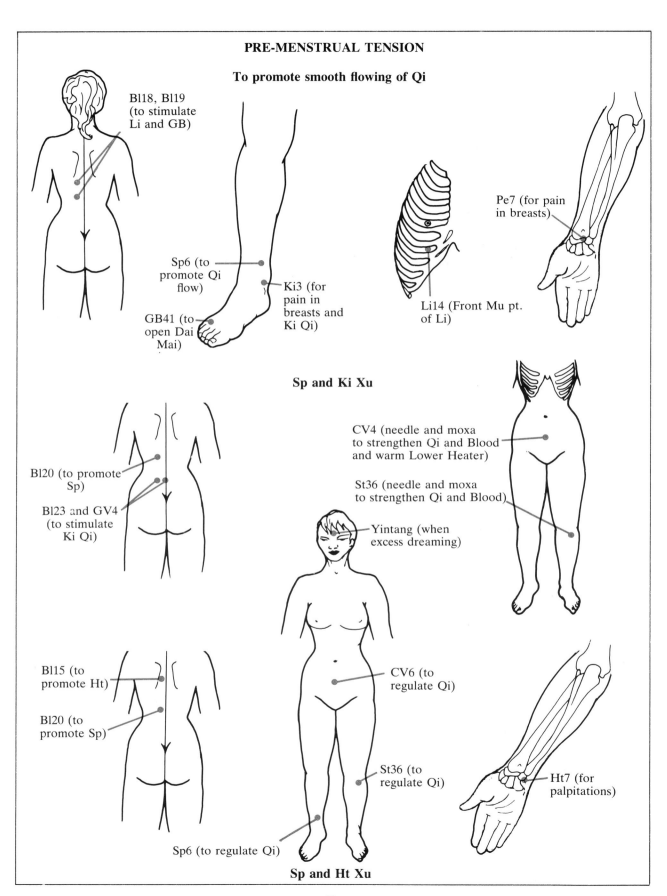

Bl18, Bl19 (to stimulate Li and GB)

Sp6 (to promote Qi flow)

Ki3 (for pain in breasts and Ki Qi)

GB41 (to open Dai Mai)

Pe7 (for pain in breasts)

Li14 (Front Mu pt. of Li)

## Sp and Ki Xu

Bl20 (to promote Sp)

Bl23 and GV4 (to stimulate Ki Qi)

CV4 (needle and moxa to strengthen Qi and Blood and warm Lower Heater)

St36 (needle and moxa to strengthen Qi and Blood)

Yintang (when excess dreaming)

Bl15 (to promote Ht)

Bl20 (to promote Sp)

CV6 (to regulate Qi)

St36 (to regulate Qi)

Ht7 (for palpitations)

Sp6 (to regulate Qi)

## Sp and Ht Xu

## Pain in Breasts

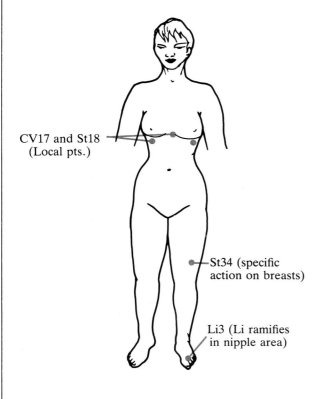

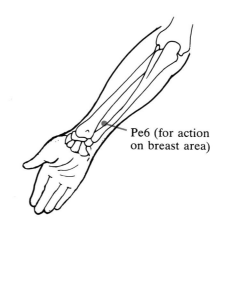

CV17 and St18
(Local pts.)

Pe6 (for action
on breast area)

St34 (specific
action on breasts)

Li3 (Li ramifies
in nipple area)

## For tension generally

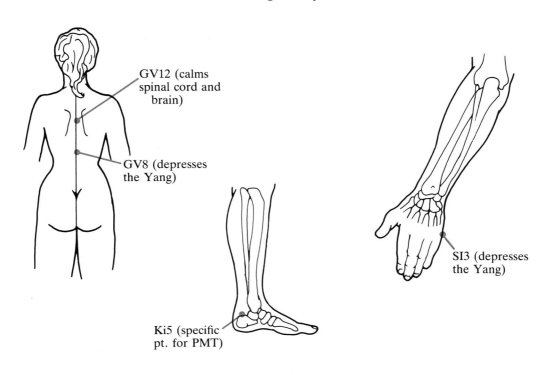

GV12 (calms
spinal cord and
brain)

GV8 (depresses
the Yang)

SI3 (depresses
the Yang)

Ki5 (specific
pt. for PMT)

# MENOPAUSAL SYMPTOMS

Before we consider the general run of menopausal symptoms, one thing must be very carefully borne in mind – all cases of post-menopausal bleeding should be treated with the utmost gravity, and *every case assumed to be due to carcinoma* until full investigations prove otherwise. Occasionally, one may get withdrawal bleeding after the administration of oestrogens, but it is very dangerous to assume that this is the case.

The major causes of post-menopausal bleeding are:
Carcinoma of the vulva, vagina, cervix, uterine body, or Fallopian tubes.
Feminizing, theca cell and granulosa cell tumours of the ovary.
Urethral caruncle; atrophic ('senile') vaginitis; vaginal ulceration from the pressure of a foreign body, such as a pessary; cervical polyp; or, in the body of the uterus, senile endometritis, polyp, submucous fibroid, mesodermal tumours, or sarcoma.

In rare cases, between the ages of 60 and 70, the endometrium thickens and menstruation recommences. This is due to an oestrogenic tumour of the ovary.

A severe case of itching of the vulva in an elderly woman may be an early sign of Leukoplakia Vulvae. As this develops the labia majora become smooth, flat and shiny, and greyish-white ('parchment') in colour, and later, fissures and warts develop. This is a pre-cancerous condition, so specialized investigations should be undertaken at an early stage.

Menopausal conditions *per se* can prove notoriously difficult to treat, as so often they are simply part of a natural senescence and simply reveal pre-existing imbalances, as it is a time of mental and energetic instability. Nevertheless, the various symptoms produced can be extremely distressing, with hot flushes and sweating attacks, indigestion and flatulence. Pains in the joints and backache are common complaints, and menopausal fibrositis and arthritis are recognized conditions. The patient is also frequently irritable and depressed.

Traditionally, in a woman the menopause starts at $7 \times 7 = 49$ years, whilst in a man the process is slower, and starts at $7 \times 8 = 56$ years to finish at $8 \times 8 = 64$ years.

It is accompanied by:
Weakness in Chong Mai
Emptiness in Ren Mai
Celestial Kwei disappears
– less concentration of energy in pelvic area
– by emptiness of blood in pelvic basin – discharges
Inner paths are cut
– by emptiness of Yin below and escape of Yang above – high colour.
Earth lines are obstructed
– by loss of menses and procreation
Ching diminishes – body withers
Infertility

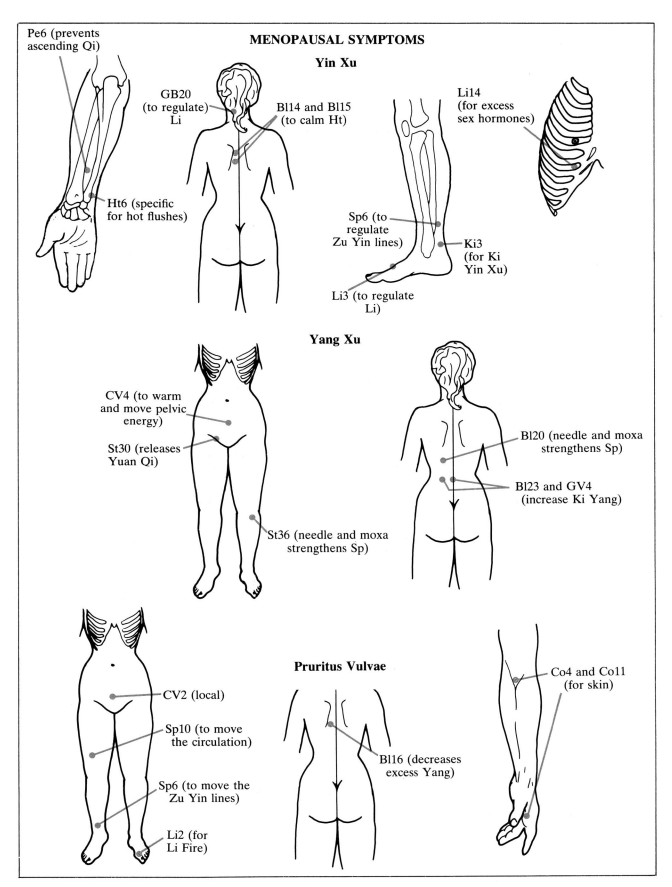

# MENOPAUSAL SYMPTOMS

## Yin Xu

Pe6 (prevents ascending Qi)

GB20 (to regulate) Li

Bl14 and Bl15 (to calm Ht)

Ht6 (specific for hot flushes)

Li14 (for excess sex hormones)

Sp6 (to regulate Zu Yin lines)

Ki3 (for Ki Yin Xu)

Li3 (to regulate Li)

## Yang Xu

CV4 (to warm and move pelvic energy)

St30 (releases Yuan Qi)

St36 (needle and moxa strengthens Sp)

Bl20 (needle and moxa strengthens Sp)

Bl23 and GV4 (increase Ki Yang)

## Pruritus Vulvae

CV2 (local)

Sp10 (to move the circulation)

Sp6 (to move the Zu Yin lines)

Li2 (for Li Fire)

Bl16 (decreases excess Yang)

Co4 and Co11 (for skin)

It is considered to present as one of two basic syndromes – either Yin Xu or Yang Xu, and to involve mainly the Liver, Kidney and Heart in the Yin Xu condition and Kidney and Spleen in the Yang Xu.

Yin Xu will present with symptoms of irritability, hot flushes, sweating, some hypertension and possibly slight vertigo, due to lack of Yin and faulty elimination of sex hormones by the Liver. One of the most important points is Ht6 (Yinxi) (the Heart Xi-Cleft point), which is invaluable in preventing the hot flushes and Yin Xu sweating, whilst we would also use Bl14 (Jueyinshu) and Bl15 (Xinshu) to calm the Heart, Sp6 (Sanyinjiao) to regulate the three Zu Yin, Li3 (Taichong) and GB20 (Fengchi) to regulate the Liver for hypertension. Also to be considered are Li14 (Qimen) to help the Liver to disperse the excess sex-hormones and possibly P6 (Neiguan), which helps to prevent the adverse ascent of Qi and will also help with vomiting and the hot flushes. Ki3 (Taixi) also is of particular value in Kidney Yin Xu.

Yang Xu will present as a general lack of Yang and weakness of Kidney Yang, with a sensitivity to cold, poor appetite, lassitude, possible oedema pedum, and diarrhoea. We will have to strengthen the function of the Spleen by needle and moxa on Bl20 (Pishu) and St36 (Zusanli); CV4 (Guanyuan) to warm and move the pelvic energy and help the Kidney, and Bl23 (Shenshu) and GV4 (Mingmen) to increase the Kidney Yang.

One point which is not used enough in menopausal conditions is St30 (Qichong). It must be remembered that this point, in conjunction with St36 (Zusanli), is part of the 'Sea of Nourishment'. It is the origin of the lower path of Chong Mai and is also, via the Spleen Divergent meridian, the lower meeting point between Stomach and Spleen. It has the effect of causing a general release of Yuan Qi in the pelvic basin, and has a specific effect in menopausal states.

A fairly common condition, usually associated with a drying up of the normal vaginal fluids, is Pruritus vulvae, traditionally ascribed to a Shi or excess condition of the Liver. The following points have proved of assistance in treating this distressing (and embarrassing!) complaint:

> CV2 (Qugu) – local.
> Bl16 (Dushu) – affects excess Yang.
> Co4 (Hegu) and Co11 (Quchi) – for the skin.
> Li2 (Xingjian) – for Liver Fire.
> Sp6 (Sanyinjiao) and Sp10 (Xuehai) – to regularize the three leg Yin and to move the circulation.

As with all conditions, however, treatment should not be initiated without prior thorough examination, to eliminate parasitic or allergic causes. Deficiencies of Vitamins A and/or B may exist, and one should always remember that there may be an untreated diabetes present. The more common cause in post-menopausal women is chronic epithelial dystrophy, which has two main origins:

(a) leukoplakia, with characteristic white patches. It does not involve the vagina but may spread beyond the vulva into the groin and around the anus, and can be pre-cancerous. Luckily it is not very common.

(b) Lichen sclerosus vel atrophicus. This is purely atrophic and does not spread beyond the vulva.

# UTERINE DISPLACEMENTS

The normal position of the uterus is that of anteversion and anteflexion, meaning that the fundus is tilted forwards towards the anterior wall of the abdomen. It is kept in position by the cardinal (or transverse cervical) ligaments from side to side and by the utero-sacral ligaments from behind, leaving the body of the uterus free to move in all directions, to expand during pregnancy, and to change its position when the bladder or rectum distends. It is supported by the round ligaments, the broad ligaments, and the pubo-cervical fascia at the front, and the pelvic floor and levatores ani from below.

Ordinarily the ligaments are in a state of relaxation and limit the normal range of the movements of the uterus. Backward displacement of the body is resisted by the round ligaments, backward displacement of the cervix by the utero-vesical ligaments, downward and forward displacements by the sacro-uterine, and lateral displacements by the broad ligaments.

The vaginal walls, being a part of the pelvic floor, also help to support the uterus, and a weakness of the walls is an indication and is a forerunner of prolapsus uteri.

The pathological changes in position are either an increase in its normal anteversion and anteflexion, retroversion, or prolapse, and may be caused by:

(a) Weakening of the ligaments from stretching during pregnancy or labour.

(b) Weakening and stretching of the muscles of the pelvic floor from the same causes.
(c) Tumours, including uterine fibroids or an ovarian tumour in the utero-vesical pouch (these will cause retroversion), or tumours lying above it which can produce exaggerated anteflexion.
(d) So-called 'congenital retroversion' – actually not strictly congenital, as it appears when the uterus grows to its normal size, but is apparently associated with a shallow anterior vaginal fornix.

## Anteflexion
As has been stated, anteversion is the normal condition. Any increase in anteflexion will normally be due to the presence of a tumour and should be referred for specialist opinion. The main symptoms are pain present over the uterus and reflected to the symphysis and lower lumbar region, and frequency caused by irritation of the bladder from pressure from the anteflexed uterus. There may also be endometritis.

## Retroversion
Generally, this is accompanied by no symptoms whatsoever, and where this is the case it is often best to disregard it, to avoid causing unnecessary apprehension for the patient.

Diagnosis is by bimanual examination either via the rectum or the vagina, and relies upon three cardinal signs:

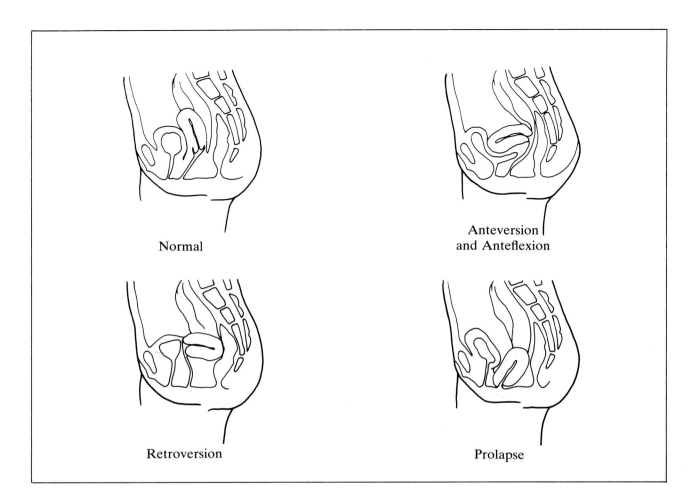

Normal

Anteversion
and Anteflexion

Retroversion

Prolapse

(i) The cervix points forward.

(ii) From either the posterior fornix or the anterior rectal wall, the body of the uterus will be felt lying in the pouch of Douglas.

(iii) The body of the uterus is not in its normal position.

Where symptoms are present, they will usually consist of:

(a) Backache, which is one of the commonest symptoms attending any displacement, but especially retroflexion. It may be a dull constant ache or it may be an actual pain, which is aggravated by muscular action and at the menstrual period, often worse in the evening after long standing during the day. A severe form of sciatica can also occur, being partly due to pressure on the sacral nerves and partly due to inflammation of the uterus (if present) extending to the nerve.

(b) Dysmenorrhoea and menorrhagia due to pelvic congestion.

(c) Dyspareunia due to pressure on prolapsed ovaries.

(d) Sterility, most likely due to lack of insemination from the forward pointing cervix.

(e) Miscarriage or habitual abortion.

Treatment would of necessity involve the manual replacement of the uterus, and either the use of a pessary to hold the uterus in place or surgical intervention, usually a ventrosuspension. The method of treatment would naturally call for referral to a consultant gynaecologist. Functional symptoms such as menorrhagia or spasmodic dysmenorrhoea respond disappointingly to surgery, but are the very ones in which acupuncture treatment is likely to prove most effective. Acupuncture is also frequently successful in strengthening the muscular and ligamentous attachments – see under the next heading.

## Uterine prolapse

This is the most common of all uterine

68

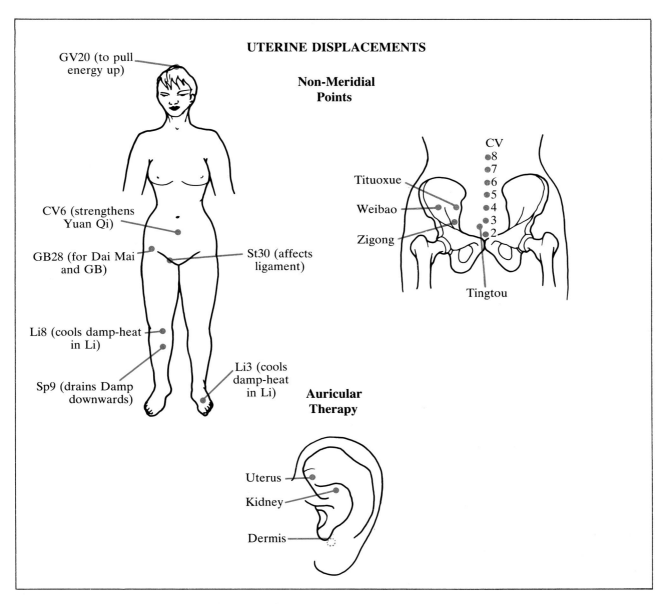

## UTERINE DISPLACEMENTS

### Non-Meridial Points

GV20 (to pull energy up)

CV6 (strengthens Yuan Qi)

GB28 (for Dai Mai and GB)

St30 (affects ligament)

Li8 (cools damp-heat in Li)

Sp9 (drains Damp downwards)

Li3 (cools damp-heat in Li)

CV
8
7
6
5
4
3
2

Tituoxue

Weibao

Zigong

Tingtou

### Auricular Therapy

Uterus

Kidney

Dermis

displacements. The main cause is a weakened pelvic floor with weakening and relaxation of the utero-sacral ligaments, and is often produced by multiple pregnancies with lack of proper postnatal care. However, anything which can produce an increase in pressure in the pelvic basin can predispose to it, whilst sudden falls or strains (particularly with a full bladder) can result in retroversion and prolapse.

Three degrees are recognized:

### Grade 1:
The uterus retroverts but does not retroflex, and it descends with sagging of the vaginal walls and, commonly, a slight degree of herniation of the bladder into the vagina.

### Grade 2:
The uterus descends into the vagina. The cervix elongates and protrudes from the vagina on straining or standing.

### Grade 3:
(Also known as procidentia). The vagina turns inside out and the entire uterus protrudes from the vulval orifice. As the uterus descends it pulls the pouch of Douglas and part of the rectum with it posteriorly (rectocoele) and the bladder anteriorly (cystocoele).

Prolapse is a frequent cause of pain and discomfort in young and middle-aged women, and although sometimes there may be a fair degree of prolapse with no untoward inconvenience, in other cases the discomfort can be considerable.

One of the major symptoms is often said to be backache, but this is usually due not to the prolapse *per se* but to the pulling on the utero-sacral ligaments exacerbating an already existing low back condition. The patient commonly complains of 'bearing-down' pains, worse during the day and better for rest, and a feeling of fullness in the vagina, sometimes 'as if there was a lump there'. Frequency of micturition, usually diurnal only, is common, and stress incontinence may be present. Sometimes there may be difficulty in complete emptying of the bladder, the patient having to press the prolapse up manually before she can complete the act. It is also common to find some form of vaginal discharge, due either to decubitus ulceration (when it may be bloodstained) or cervical congestion or erosion, whilst constipation is often complained of – possibly because of the bulging of the rectum into the posterior vaginal wall, which may cause difficulty with evacuation.

Acupuncture will give good results with Grades 1 and 2. Where Grade 3 is concerned the patient will necessarily need to be referred to a specialist.

The traditional Chinese approach postulates the trouble as being due mainly to weak or 'sunken' Qi of the Middle Heater, where the Irregular Vessels Chong Mai and Ren Mai fail to keep the uterus in place. Alternatively, Damp-Heat moving into the Lower Heater may cause the uterus to fall.

Weak Qi symptoms are: pallor, sensitivity to cold, lassitude, palpitations, and frequency.

The symptoms of Damp-Heat are: irritability, bitter taste in the mouth, a depressed feeling in the chest, and blockage in the stomach.

The usual points in use are GV20 (Baihui), St30 (Qichong), GB28 (Weidao) and Sp6 (Sanyinjiao). Better results can often be achieved if GB28 is stimulated electrically.

Secondary points are: CV6 (Qihai), Sp9 (Yinlingquan), Li3 (Taichong) and Li8 (Ququan).

GB28 (Weidao) is used as the intersection of Dai Mai and the Gall Bladder meridian – insert into the broad uterine ligament, obliquely, medially and inferiorly, 1.5 to 2 cun.

St30 (Qichong) is over the Fallopian ligament, and is the reunion of Chong Mai with the Stomach and Gall Bladder meridians.

GV20 (Baihui) is the reunion of Du Mai and the Bladder meridian.

CV6 (Qihai) strengthens the Yuan Qi.

Li3 (Taichong) and Li8 (Ququan) are used to cool heat.

Sp9 (Yinlingquan) drains excess Damp downwards.

Quite spectacular results may be obtained by the use of non-meridial point Zigong, situated 3 cun laterally to CV3 (Zhongji). The patient is placed in the supine position, preferably with the head below the level of the feet, and the point is stimulated strongly. The uterus will often be felt returning to its corrected position almost immediately – unfortunately, the correction is only maintained for a few hours but, logically, one cannot expect a simple intervention such as this to correct a long-standing weakness of the whole pelvic basin, and further steps must necessarily be taken.

Other non-meridial points to consider are Tituoxue (4 cun lateral to CV4 (Guanyuan)) used more especially for ovarian troubles, and possibly Weibao (in the depression below and medial to the anterior superior iliac spine, aproximately on the level of CV4) or Tingtou (½ cun below Ki12 (Dabe)).

Auricular points used are Uterus, Kidney, and Dermis (Sub-Cortex).

It must be realized that in all cases the prolapsed uterus must be reduced before acupuncture treatment is commenced. After treatment, the patient should be instructed to lie in the foetal position for twenty to thirty minutes.

# INFERTILITY

When dealing with the question of infertility, the first thing to bear in mind is that 'it takes two to tango', and it is always essential to eliminate any deficiency on the part of the male partner before querying the female role.

The chief causes where the man is concerned are weakness in the sperm, general impotence, or premature ejaculation. Weakness in the sperm can be verified by having a sperm count done – if there is a low count, the traditional approach is to advise the patient to 'thicken the sperm' by abstaining from intercourse for a long enough time to allow the body to 'recuperate the essence', and generally to lead as healthy a life as possible. Weakness in the sperm and a degree of impotence can also be attributed to general debility, either from an unhealthy lifestyle, illness, or just old age. The advice here is to build up the energy, again by adopting a healthy dietetic and exercise regime, using herbs such as ginseng and Astragalus, and acupuncture formulae to build up the general vitality – such points as Bl23 (Shenshu), GV4 (Mingmen), St36 (Zusanli) and CV4 (Guanyuan) will all help, with moxa of GV20 (Baihui) to raise the Yang and additional points Ki3 (Taixi), Sp6 (Sanyinjiao), CV12 (Zhongwan), CV6 (Qihai) and GV14 (Dazhui) selected from, preferably with moxa on heated needle.

Overwork and general mental strain can cause impotence by injuring the heart and spleen, with concomitant symptoms of restless sleep, irritability and loss of appetite. In such a case we would select from the above points to strengthen the general energy, but also add Bl15 (Xinshu), Ht7 (Shenmen), and possibly P6 (Neiguan) to nourish the heart. A general weakness in the pelvic basin may occasionally be caused by a build-up of Damp-Heat, particularly in the Liver channel. This will call for treatment to assist the liver and spleen and to disperse the Damp-Heat. Because it is a 'hot' condition moxa is contra-indicated, so we stimulate Sp6 (Sanyinjiao), Bl23 (Shenshu), Bl19 (Danshu), Li5 (Ligou – luo point of Liver), and CV4 (Guanyuan), possibly adding Li3 (Taichong) and GB34 (Yanglingquan).

Premature ejaculation may sometimes be the cause of a failure to conceive due to an insufficiency of semen actually entering into the womb. It is traditionally regarded as being a 'False Yang' – an excess of Yang due to an underlying deficiency of Yin which is unable to hold the Yang back. Fundamentally it is a deep-seated problem, with roots in both the psychological and physical structure of the man. Treatment consists in building up the Kidney Yin, best achieved by endeavouring to get the patient to 'slow down' both mentally and physically, and by the judicious use of herbs and diet. Acupuncture can help by a careful combination of treatments to build the basic pelvic energy – Ki3 (Taixi), Bl23 (Shenshu), CV4 (Guanyuan), etc.

Particular points for impotence in general are CV3 (Zhingji), for weak erection and involuntary emission, and Ki2 (Rangu).

Insofar as the female is concerned, sterility is regarded as being either primary or secondary. Primary infertility may be due to a number of factors, one of the most obvious of which would be an intact hymen, abnormality of the vagina, cervix or uterus, blockage of the Fallopian tubes, salpingitis, or some abnormality of the ovaries causing a hormonal imbalance or possible anovulatory cycles.

Secondary sterility refers to instances when a woman who has previously been fertile ceases to be capable of pregnancy – usually as the result of uterine infection.

The general state of health will also have an effect, with diseases such as diabetes or nephritis or disorders such as obesity or thyroid deficiency, not to mention the general diminution of fertility due to age (fertility generally being considered as diminishing after the age of 35) all having to be considered.

Tests for tubal patency will necessarily have to be carried out in a hospital, involving either laparoscopy or hysterosalpingography, and may require surgical intervention for correction.

TCM enumerates twelve possible causes, some of which correspond to the Western concepts, others which take a more energetic viewpoint:

Abnormality of the uterus (retroversion etc.)
Stagnant blood in the Lower Heater.
Deficiency in Dai Mai.
Excess in Dai Mai.
Cold in the uterus.
Cold in the pelvic basin.
Heat in the pelvic basin.
Imbalance in the circulation of fluids.
Obesity.
Emaciation.
Weakness.
Jealousy.

Malposition of the uterus has been dealt with previously. Excess or deficiency of Dai Mai (the 'Girdle Vessel') would be treated appropriately with points such as GB26 (Daimai), GB41 (Linqi), also GV3 (Yaoyangguan) to bring Yang down and out, St37 (Shangjuxu) for excess in the upper part of the body, St39 (Xiajuxu) for deficiency in the lower part of the body, CV4 (Guanyuan) and CV6 (Qihai), as the symptoms require.

Stagnant blood in the Lower Heater is often emotional in origin, being the result of retardation of Liver Qi. It will often show up as a patch of dirty browny-black fur at the very back of the tongue – interestingly enough, the Mu point for the Triple Heater as a whole – CV5 (Shimen) – is often said to be contra-indicated in women as its use may cause infertility! But the Mu point for the Lower Heater – CV7 (Yinjiao) can be of assistance in this condition. Other points of use are CV6 (Qihai), Sp10 (Xuehai), Li14 (Qimen), and possibly Sp8 (Diji), all to produce a free-flowing of the blood.

'Cold in the uterus' will exhibit signs of deficiency of blood, and we therefore need to tone the blood and warm the area – moxa Bl20 (Pishu), Bl23 (Shenshu), Sp6 (Sanyinjiao), Sp8 (Diji) and CV4 (Guanyuan) can be a useful approach.

Cold in the lower abdomen is usually a Kidney Yang Xu – moxa Bl23 (Shensu), GV4 (Mingmen), CV4 (Guanyuan), Sp6 (Sanyinjiao), and St36 (Zusanli).

Heat in the lower abdomen is usually a false fire due to Kidney Yin Xu, and calls for stimulation (not moxa) of possibly Bl23 (Shenshu), GV4 (Mingmen), Ki3 (Taixi), CV6 (Qihai), Sp6 (Sanyinjiao), and Bl38 (Gaohuangshu), possibly with the addition of GV14 (Dazhui) to bring the Yang up and out.

Imbalance in the circulation of fluids often goes hand in hand with obesity, the latter being due to the accumulation of fluid. We therefore need to disperse the fluids and at the same time strengthen the body's metabolism, via Bl20 (Pishu), Bl21 (Weishu), St36 (Zusanli), St40 (Fenglong), CV12 (Zhongwan) possibly alternated with Ki6 (Zhaohai), Lu7 (Lieque) and CV9 (Shuifen) for fluid control via Ren Mai and the Yinqiao.

Emaciation, often associated with a drying up of the fluids, is often due to a condition of internal fire, in the majority of cases brought on by an excess of Liver Yang and a deficiency of Kidney Yin. The ultimate diagnosis will naturally depend upon an assessment of the patient's overall energic balance.

Two useful non-meridial points in all cases of infertility are Xingqixue (with the navel as the apex of an equilaterial triangle, each side 3 cun

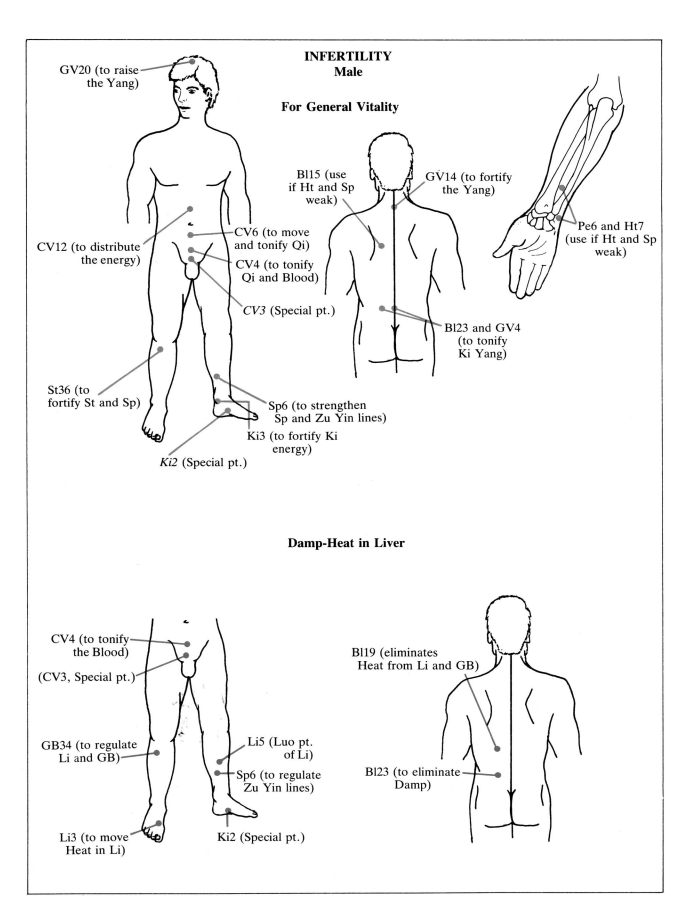

**INFERTILITY**
**Male**

**For General Vitality**

GV20 (to raise the Yang)

CV12 (to distribute the energy)

CV6 (to move and tonify Qi)

CV4 (to tonify Qi and Blood)

*CV3* (Special pt.)

St36 (to fortify St and Sp)

Sp6 (to strengthen Sp and Zu Yin lines)

Ki3 (to fortify Ki energy)

*Ki2* (Special pt.)

Bl15 (use if Ht and Sp weak)

GV14 (to fortify the Yang)

Bl23 and GV4 (to tonify Ki Yang)

Pe6 and Ht7 (use if Ht and Sp weak)

**Damp-Heat in Liver**

CV4 (to tonify the Blood)

(CV3, Special pt.)

GB34 (to regulate Li and GB)

Li5 (Luo pt. of Li)

Sp6 (to regulate Zu Yin lines)

Li3 (to move Heat in Li)

Ki2 (Special pt.)

Bl19 (eliminates Heat from Li and GB)

Bl23 (to eliminate Damp)

73

# INFERTILITY
## Female

### Trouble in Dai Mai

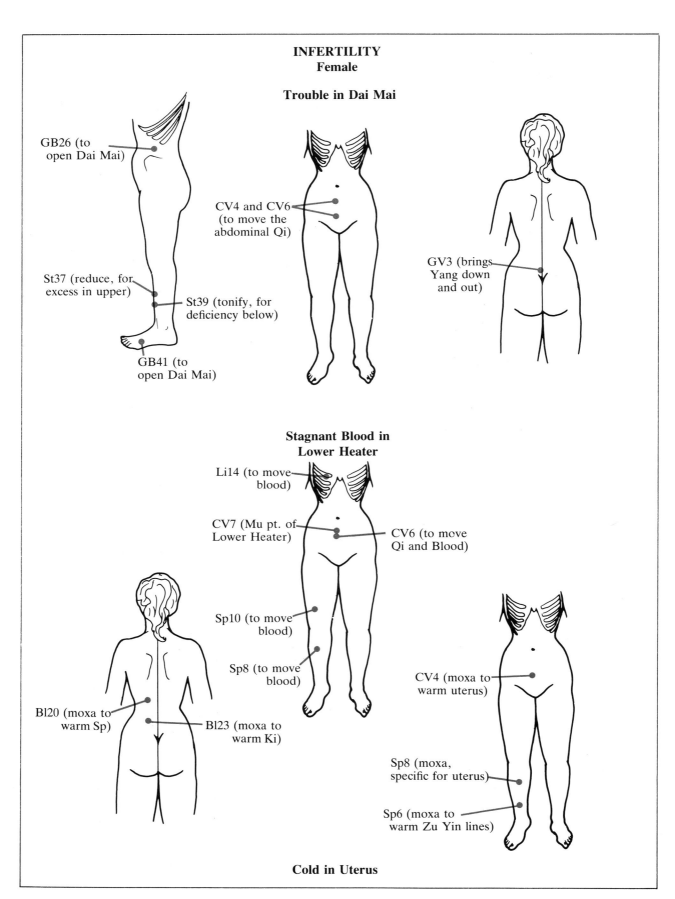

GB26 (to open Dai Mai)

CV4 and CV6 (to move the abdominal Qi)

GV3 (brings Yang down and out)

St37 (reduce, for excess in upper)

St39 (tonify, for deficiency below)

GB41 (to open Dai Mai)

### Stagnant Blood in Lower Heater

Li14 (to move blood)

CV7 (Mu pt. of Lower Heater)

CV6 (to move Qi and Blood)

Sp10 (to move blood)

Sp8 (to move blood)

Bl20 (moxa to warm Sp)

Bl23 (moxa to warm Ki)

CV4 (moxa to warm uterus)

Sp8 (moxa, specific for uterus)

Sp6 (moxa to warm Zu Yin lines)

**Cold in Uterus**

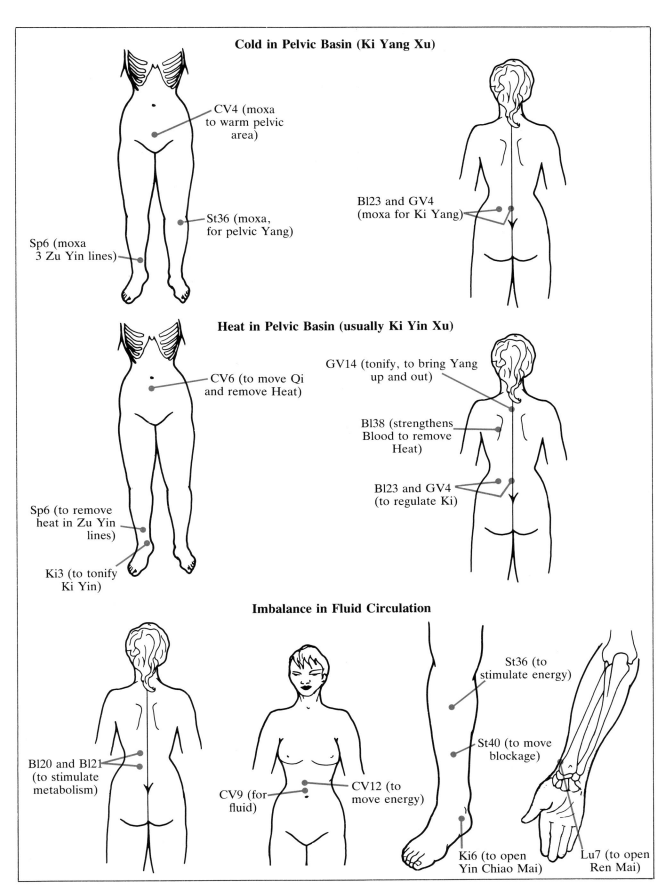

**Cold in Pelvic Basin (Ki Yang Xu)**

CV4 (moxa to warm pelvic area)

St36 (moxa, for pelvic Yang)

Sp6 (moxa 3 Zu Yin lines)

Bl23 and GV4 (moxa for Ki Yang)

**Heat in Pelvic Basin (usually Ki Yin Xu)**

CV6 (to move Qi and remove Heat)

GV14 (tonify, to bring Yang up and out)

Bl38 (strengthens Blood to remove Heat)

Bl23 and GV4 (to regulate Ki)

Sp6 (to remove heat in Zu Yin lines)

Ki3 (to tonify Ki Yin)

**Imbalance in Fluid Circulation**

Bl20 and Bl21 (to stimulate metabolism)

CV9 (for fluid)

CV12 (to move energy)

St36 (to stimulate energy)

St40 (to move blockage)

Ki6 (to open Yin Chiao Mai)

Lu7 (to open Ren Mai)

apex of an equilaterial triangle, each side 3 cun long, the point is at either end of the base line)

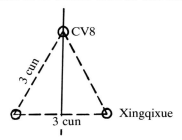

and Zigong (3 cun lateral to CV3 (Zhongji).

Infertility is not always the easiest of conditions to treat, and it is of course essential that the underlying cause be discovered before any attempt at treatment is instigated. Although occasionally almost 'miraculous' cures have been obtained with acupuncture, it is usually advisable to warn the patient that a long course of treatment may be required.

# Part Two:
# Disorders of pregnancy

# DISORDERS OF PREGNANCY

Every acupuncturist will be aware that, because of its profound effect upon the energetic balance of the body, acupuncture during pregnancy should be approached with extreme caution. Unless the practitioner is extremely experienced, a safe rule is that at no time during pregnancy should any point below the umbilicus be punctured, and after the fifth month no point upon the stomach. The two points Sp6 (Sanyin-jiao) and Co4 (Hegu) are at all times strongly contra-indicated – indeed, Co4 is sometimes termed 'The Great Eliminator' so the barring of this point is understandable. Any treatment to induce sweating is also undesirable, as it tends to dry up the body fluids and injure the Yang and Qi.

The only treatment which has been recommended (by Flaws, 'The Path of Pregnancy') is the stimulation of Ki9 (Zhubin) at the end of the third and sixth months. Ki9 is the Xi-Cleft point of the Yin Wei Mai, and it is claimed that it minimizes the transmission of toxins from mother to child, increases the health of the baby and its resistance to disease, and also tonifies the mother's Qi.

# MORNING SICKNESS

Although this is a very common condition, when it persists beyond the first trimester it is called hyperemesis gravidum, and is regarded as being serious.

Morning sickness is traditionally thought of as being due to hyperactivity of the Liver, deficiency of Stomach/Spleen, and accumulation of Damp-Phlegm.

It can manifest as:

## (a) Liver Qi rising upwards
This gives acid vomiting, regurgitation and belching, a bitter taste in the mouth and congestion in the chest. The pulse is fast and wiry and the tongue often has a heavy, sticky coat.

*Treatment:* St 36 (Zusanli), P6 (Neiguan), CV12 (Zhongwan), St44 (Neiting) and Li2 (Xingjian).

## (b) Yang Qi rebelling upwards
With this there is thirst for water but vomiting it up after drinking, dizziness, tinnitus, insomnia, palpitations, and chest congestion. The pulse is generally rapid and weak, whilst the tongue has little or no fur and is possibly reddish.

*Treatment:* St36 (Zusanli), P6 (Neiguan), CV12 (Zhongwan), Sp4 (Gongsun) and Ki3 (Taixi).

## (c) Phlegm-Damp obstructing the Stomach
Symptoms of acid regurgitation and vomiting of watery substance, dizziness, palpitations, congestion in the chest; food seems tasteless. Pulse wiry and slippery, the tongue is pale with a whitish, sticky coating.

*Treatment:* St36 (Zusanli), P6 Neiguan), CV12 (Zhongwan), Sp4 (Gongsun), St40 (Fenglong), moxa CV17 (Shanzhong). Can add Bl20 (Pishu) and Bl21 (Weishu).

Auricular points for the general condition could consist of Liver, Stomach, Shenmen and Sympathetic. It will be noticed that all the treatments given above include the point P6 (Neiguan) – this may be regarded as almost a specific for all cases involving vomiting.

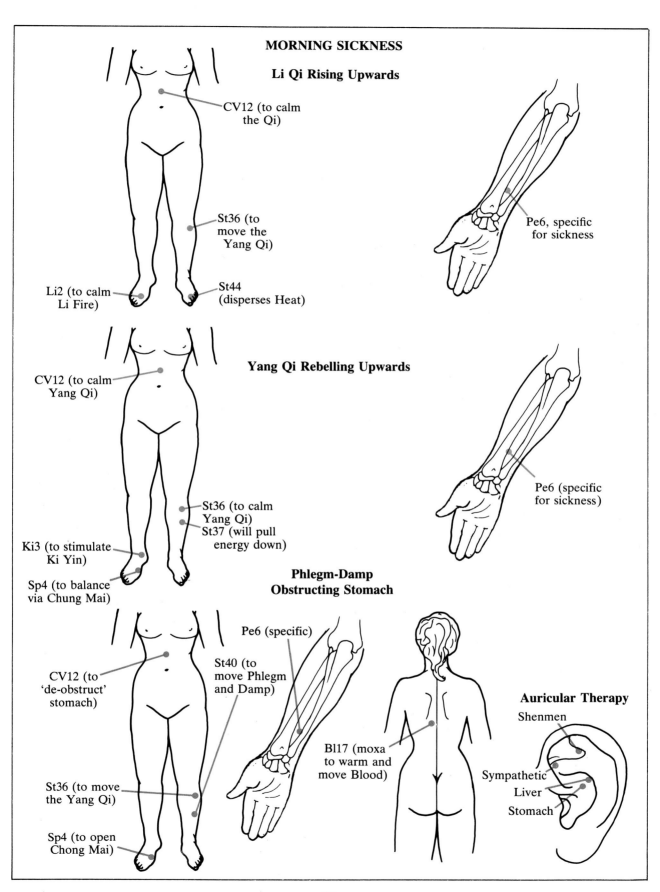

**MORNING SICKNESS**

**Li Qi Rising Upwards**

CV12 (to calm the Qi)

St36 (to move the Yang Qi)

Li2 (to calm Li Fire)

St44 (disperses Heat)

Pe6, specific for sickness

**Yang Qi Rebelling Upwards**

CV12 (to calm Yang Qi)

St36 (to calm Yang Qi)

St37 (will pull energy down)

Ki3 (to stimulate Ki Yin)

Sp4 (to balance via Chung Mai)

Pe6 (specific for sickness)

**Phlegm-Damp Obstructing Stomach**

Pe6 (specific)

St40 (to move Phlegm and Damp)

CV12 (to 'de-obstruct' stomach)

St36 (to move the Yang Qi)

Sp4 (to open Chong Mai)

Bl17 (moxa to warm and move Blood)

**Auricular Therapy**

Shenmen

Sympathetic

Liver

Stomach

# ABDOMINAL PAIN DURING PREGNANCY

The use of acupuncture is generally considered to be contra-indicated in this context, and reliance should be placed upon the use of herbs.

There are four possible causes which we should consider:

## (a) Attack by Cold

The patient feels cold inside, with a possible feeling of swelling in the womb. The face may be puffy and there may be loose stools. The pulse is deep and wiry and the tongue pale with a thin white, sometimes sticky, coat.

The patient should be instructed to dress warmly, and warming herbs and foods prescribed.

## (b) Deficiency of Qi and Blood

Presents with a dragging pain over the lumbar and abdominal areas, with a bearing-down sensation. The patient is listless, with a poor appetite, withered complexion, dyspnoea, possibly dizziness and palpitations. The pulse is either thready and weak or large and hollow, the tongue pale with a thin whitish coating.

These patients need rest and plenty of nourishing food, plus herbal supplements such as the Ba Zhong Yi Qi Tang formula.

## (c) Qi Stagnation

This gives congestion and pain in the abdomen and thorax, with abdominal distension, borborygmus, general depression and irritability, thirst, concentrated urine and dry faeces, and a bitter taste in the mouth. The pulse is wiry, the tongue coating thin and sticky.

Warm compresses to the abdomen may help to remove the stagnation. (Warm – *not* hot!)

## (d) Stagnation of food

The patient has a feeling of fullness in the epigastrium, regurgitations with reduced appetite, and foul stools. If from Wind-Cold, there will also be pains in the joints and headaches, possibly with a fever. The tongue will have a sticky white coat.

# OEDEMA DURING PREGNANCY

This is naturally due to an accumulation of fluid, and may be caused by either a failure of the spleen to transform and transport the blood and fluids, weakness of the kidneys leading to failure to excrete the impure fluids, or to stagnation of Qi. Acupuncture can be used to correct the malfunction but, as has been said earlier, in the prevailing condition of pregnancy must be used with the greatest caution and only be an experienced practitioner.

Oedema due to *Deficiency of the Spleen* usually occurs in the earlier stages of pregnancy, and presents with a generalized oedema, especially of the face, a sallow complexion, cold limbs, a lack of taste, lack of appetite with general weakness, watery stools containing undigested food, scanty urination and, in severe cases, some mental disturbance and vertigo. The pulse is deep, hollow and slippery, the tongue pale with a thin white coating.

Treatment would obviously concentrate upon correcting the spleen deficiency, by stimulating Bl20 (Pishu), Bl21 (Weishu), Sp5 (Shangqui), Sp9 (Yinlingquan), CV12 (Zhongwan), and the special point for water metabolism – CV9 (Shuifen).

Occurring later in pregnancy is *Kidney Deficiency*, again presenting as a general oedema especially of the face, which will tend to be slightly more greyish in appearance. There will be aches in the lumbar region and possibly abdominal distension, dyspnoea, and palpitations. The pulse is frequently retarded and slightly tight or sunken, the tongue again pale with a thin white coat, slightly slippery.

To treat, we must stimulate the kidneys, with Bl23 (Shenshu), Ki3 (Taixi), Ki7 (Fului), GV4 (Mingmen), and possibly Bl28 (Pangguanshu) as the Back-Shu point of the bladder.

*Stagnation of Qi* occurs in the last half of pregnancy, and first manifests in the feet and then spreads up the legs to the waist. It is better on first rising and after being rested with the legs raised, but gets worse with weight-bearing until it actually interferes with walking. Occasionally there may be a yellowish fluid formed between the toes. With the general retardation of Qi there will be abdominal distension and congestion in the chest, a lack of appetite and a feeling of depression. The pulse will be deep, wiry and slippery, and the tongue will have a thick, greasy coating.

To move the Qi, Li13 (Zhangmen), Sp9 (Yinlingquan), GB34 (Yanglingquan), Li3 (Taichong), Bl22 (Sanjiaoshu) and Bl28 (Pangguanshu) are typical.

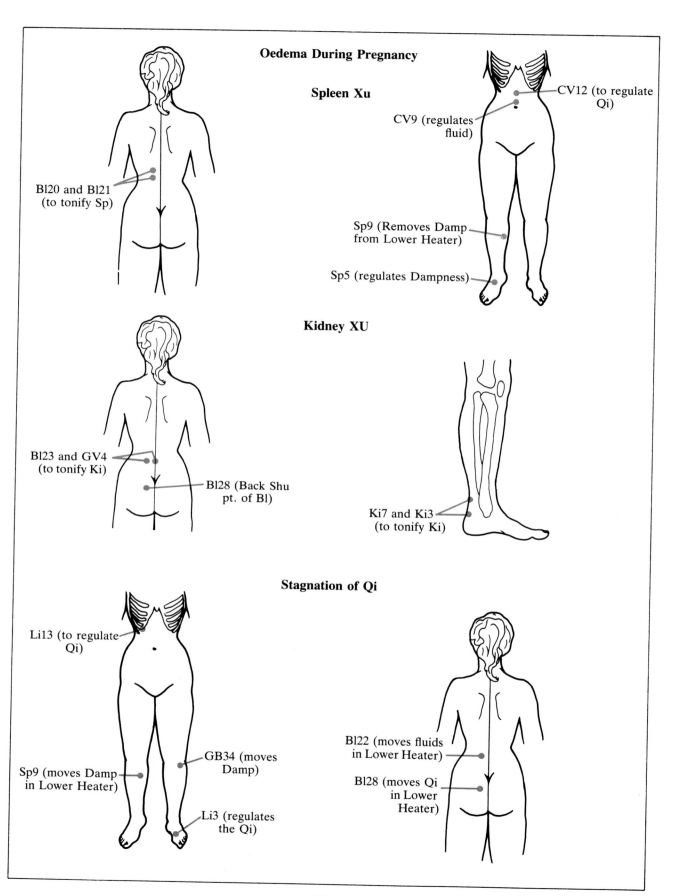

**Oedema During Pregnancy**

**Spleen Xu**

Bl20 and Bl21 (to tonify Sp)

CV12 (to regulate Qi)

CV9 (regulates fluid)

Sp9 (Removes Damp from Lower Heater)

Sp5 (regulates Dampness)

**Kidney XU**

Bl23 and GV4 (to tonify Ki)

Bl28 (Back Shu pt. of Bl)

Ki7 and Ki3 (to tonify Ki)

**Stagnation of Qi**

Li13 (to regulate Qi)

Sp9 (moves Damp in Lower Heater)

GB34 (moves Damp)

Li3 (regulates the Qi)

Bl22 (moves fluids in Lower Heater)

Bl28 (moves Qi in Lower Heater)

# ECLAMPSIA GRAVIDARUM

Eclampsia is one of the most serious complications of pregnancy, particularly if occurring during the puerperium, although it may occur either before, during or after labour.

It is characterized by severe convulsive seizures, similar to those occuring in uraemia, and is usually associated with high blood pressure and albuminuria. Regular monitoring of these two factors during pregnancy is therefore an essential feature of its prevention. If eclampsia persists for more than two or three weeks it is usual to terminate the pregnancy or perform a caesarian section, because if albuminuria continues for longer than this permanent damage to the kidneys may ensue.

The TCM syndromes are ascribed mainly to a condition of exhaustion of blood, leading to a deficiency of Yin, which in turn will present a picture of false Yang.

The basic picture of *Blood Deficiency* will lead to stagnation of Qi and the accumulation of Phlegm. There will be some obesity or oedema, possibly palpitations and dizziness, a 'cold' appearance, dyspnoea, a rattling of phlegm in the throat, and spasmodic cramping in the hands and feet. The pulse will be fine, rapid and slippery, the tongue pale, with little or no fur.

The principles of treatment would be to nourish the blood, move the Qi, and remove the phlegm, so points would be selected to achieve these objectives:

> e.g. Bl17 (Geshu), Bl20 (Pishu), Bl38
> (Gaohuangshu), Sp8 (Diji), Bl15 (Xinshu) for blood,
> GB34 (Yanglingquan), CV6 (Qihai), CV17 (Shanzhong), St36 (Zusanli), Bl15 (Xinshu) and Bl18 (Ganshu) to move the Qi, and
> St40 (Fenglong), Lu9 (Taiyuan), Sp9 (Yinlingquan) and Bl22 (Sanjiaoshu) to remove the phlegm
>
> could all be points from which to select the prescription.

Blood deficiency can be complicated with Wind Heat, or Heat in the Liver. In these instances the symptoms will change – if the blood deficiency is still paramount the complexion will be pale, but if the Liver Fire comes into excess the complexion will be reddish. There will be blurred vision, dizziness, palpitations, and anxiety accompanied by depression and tiredness, constipation with dry stools, possibly tidal fever, whilst the attack itself will bring on sudden fainting with crampy twitching of all the limbs. The pulse will be wiry, rapid, and either thready or forceful, the tongue red with a thin, dusty, yellowish coating.

Treatment to improve the blood and reduce the liver heat could utilize such points as Bl17 (Geshu), Bl20 (Pishu), Bl23 (Shenshu), Ki3 (Taixi), Li2 (Xingjian), GB20 (Fengchi) and GB37 (Guangming).

It is also possible for the syndrome of *Hot Blood* associated with *Wind* to present itself. In

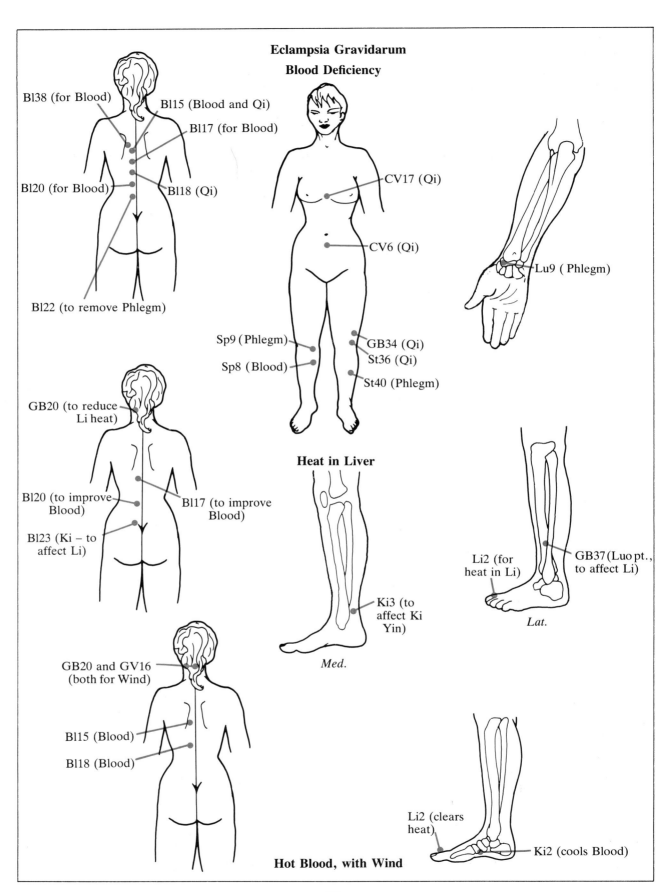

# Eclampsia Gravidarum

## Blood Deficiency

Bl38 (for Blood)

Bl15 (Blood and Qi)

Bl17 (for Blood)

Bl20 (for Blood)

Bl18 (Qi)

Bl22 (to remove Phlegm)

CV17 (Qi)

CV6 (Qi)

Lu9 ( Phlegm)

Sp9 (Phlegm)

Sp8 (Blood)

GB34 (Qi)

St36 (Qi)

St40 (Phlegm)

GB20 (to reduce Li heat)

Bl20 (to improve Blood)

Bl17 (to improve Blood)

Bl23 (Ki – to affect Li)

## Heat in Liver

Ki3 (to affect Ki Yin)

*Med.*

Li2 (for heat in Li)

GB37 (Luo pt., to affect Li)

*Lat.*

GB20 and GV16 (both for Wind)

Bl15 (Blood)

Bl18 (Blood)

Li2 (clears heat)

Ki2 (cools Blood)

## Hot Blood, with Wind

this case the attack is extremely acute, with sudden syncope, a flushed face, tetanic contractures and epigastric pain or vomiting. The pulse is wiry, rapid and slippery, the tongue red.

Suitable points could include Bl15 (Xinshu), Bl18 (Ganshu), GV16 (Fengfu), GB20 (Fengchi), Ki2 (Rangu), and Li2 (Xingjian).

It must be stressed that, thankfully, eclampsia is far less common nowadays than it used to be, thanks to careful monitoring of the blood pressure and albumin levels during the course of pregnancy, and it is not only unlikely but also undesirable that the acupuncturist should be called upon to treat this condition, except in an emergency where no specialist advice or services are available.

Early albuminuria usually calls for insistence upon bed rest, plenty of fluids such as lemonade and glucose, and drastic reduction in the protein intake.

# VAGINAL BLEEDING

Vaginal bleeding during pregnancy should not be regarded lightly, as any excessive loss of blood can seriously interfere with the nourishment of the foetus. As with abdominal pain, acupuncture is not generally advisable, and unless in exceptional circumstances the practitioner should prefer the use of herbs or other alternative treatment.

One of the commonest causes is *Deficiency of Spleen*. The leakage is naturally due to inability of the spleen to fulfil its function of holding the blood, but there will be a concomitant weakness of Qi giving signs of Cold and deficient Yang – a sallow complexion, general weakness and lack of energy, congestion in the chest, and loose stools. The tongue is pale and flabby with a thin white coat, and the pulse is weak.

The usual points to stimulate the Stomach/ Spleen are selected, such as Bl20 (Pishu), Bl21 (Weishu), St36 (Zusanli) and Sp1 (Yinbai). GV20 (Baihui) for the general Yang could also be considered.

Other causes are Wind Heat and Hot Blood.

## Wind Heat

This gives vertigo, a bitter taste in the mouth. The patient feels hot but looks cold, and is thirsty, with concentrated urine. The pulse is floating and rapid, the tongue has a thin white coating.

Dispersal points are the ones used for such a condition: Si1 (Shaoze), Co1 (Shangyang), GB20 (Fengchi), Co11 (Quchi), Ki10 (Tingu), Li8 (Ququan) etc.

## Hot Blood

This gives a profuse, dark red discharge. The condition often comes from Liver weakness, which leads to excess blood in circulation with a tendency for it to leave the vessels, so there may also be reddish skin eruptions or rashes. There could be irritability, possibly heartburn and abdominal pain. The pulse is wiry and rapid, the tongue has a thin, sticky coating.

Points to cool the blood include Sp10 (Xuehai), P3 (Quze), and Bl54 (Weizhong), whilst Bl15 (Xinshu) and Bl20 (Pishu) will strengthen the blood. For the liver weakness, Bl18 (Ganshu) can be added.

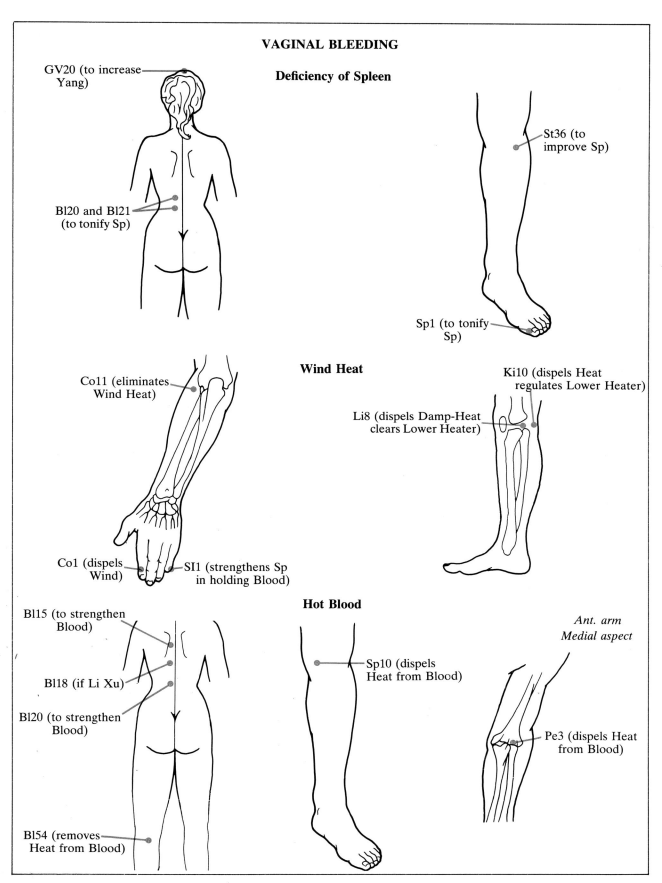

# VAGINAL BLEEDING

**Deficiency of Spleen**

GV20 (to increase Yang)

Bl20 and Bl21 (to tonify Sp)

St36 (to improve Sp)

Sp1 (to tonify Sp)

**Wind Heat**

Co11 (eliminates Wind Heat)

Ki10 (dispels Heat regulates Lower Heater)

Li8 (dispels Damp-Heat clears Lower Heater)

Co1 (dispels Wind)

SI1 (strengthens Sp in holding Blood)

**Hot Blood**

Bl15 (to strengthen Blood)

Bl18 (if Li Xu)

Bl20 (to strengthen Blood)

Bl54 (removes Heat from Blood)

Sp10 (dispels Heat from Blood)

*Ant. arm*
*Medial aspect*

Pe3 (dispels Heat from Blood)

# DYSURIA DURING PREGNANCY

It is almost to be expected that with the enlargement in size of the gravid uterus a certain amount of downward pressure would be exerted upon the bladder. As a rule this interference with normal bladder function is minimal, and causes only transient disturbance when the intra-abdominal pressure is increased by such acts as coughing or sneezing. However, if for some reason the uterus fails to be properly supported, the pressure on the bladder will be increased, and dysuria will result. In some rare cases complete anuria can occur and this, particularly during pregnancy, can be critical, and catheterisation may be necessary.

The usual TCM reason given for the lack of support is that it is due to a weakness of Qi, traditionally due to weakness in the Middle Heater. As repeatedly said before, treatment by acupuncture should be given only as a last resort, as any interference with the energic patterns during pregnancy can be highly dangerous.

There are four main syndromes recognized.
(a) Qi deficiency
(b) Kidney deficiency
(c) Damp-Heat in the Bladder
(d) Stagnation of Qi

## (a) Deficiency of Qi
This presents with either frequent, scanty urine, or with retention. The patient has a pallid complexion, with a feeling of heaviness in the head, possibly vertigo, possibly palpitations. There is general tiredness and weakness, with dyspnoea, and probably some lower abdominal distension. The pulse is weak and slippery, the tongue pale with a thin whitish coat.

Acupuncture of the more usual abdominal points such as CV4 (Guanyuan) or CV6 (Qihai) is naturally strongly contra-indicated, and emphasis is placed upon the Back-Shu points: Bl13 (Faishu), Bl20 (Pishu), Bl21 (Weishu), Bl23 (Shenshu) and Bl28 (Pangguangshu).

## (b) Deficiency of Kidney
Will start with difficult but frequent urination, followed by retention and anuria. There will be abdominal distension and a generalized tendency for oedema in the face, body, and limbs. The patient will have a darkish complexion, general weakness with aches in the lumbar area, vertigo, loose watery stools, and a general aversion to cold. The pulse will be deepish, and either slow or slippery and weak. The tongue will be pale with a thin white sticky coat.

The principle of warming the Kidney Yang is adhered to, with Ki3 (Taixi), Ki7 (Fului) and Bl23 (Shenshu), whilst to transform the fluids and Qi we use Bl22 (Sanjiaoshu) and Bl28 (Pangguangshu).

## (c) Damp Heat in the Bladder
This can simulate cystitis to start with, but proceeds into retention. The urine is short and concentrated, with a feeling of heat inside the body and abdominal distension. There may be a

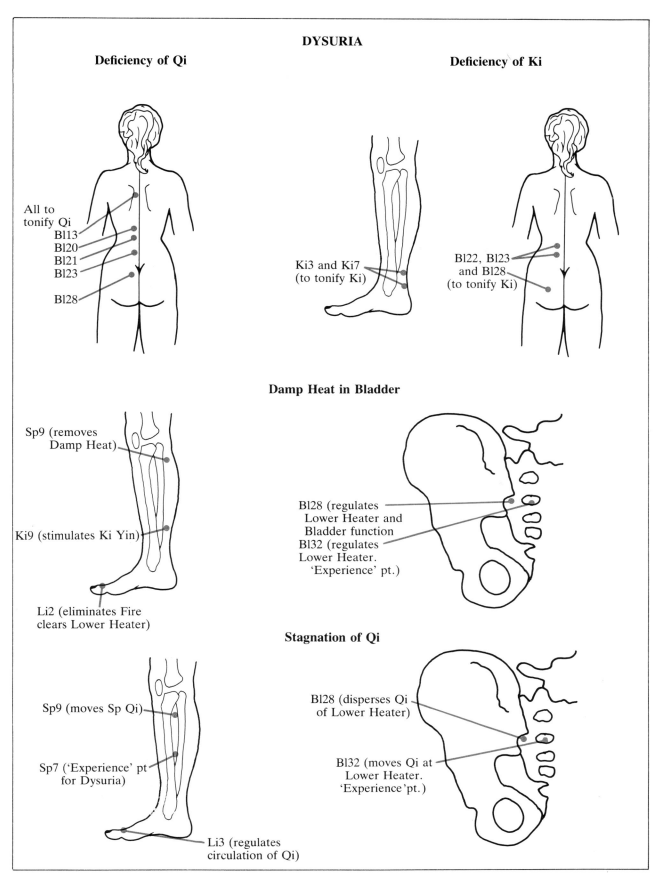

# DYSURIA

**Deficiency of Qi**

All to
tonify Qi

Bl13
Bl20
Bl21
Bl23

Bl28

**Deficiency of Ki**

Ki3 and Ki7
(to tonify Ki)

Bl22, Bl23
and Bl28
(to tonify Ki)

**Damp Heat in Bladder**

Sp9 (removes
Damp Heat)

Ki9 (stimulates Ki Yin)

Li2 (eliminates Fire
clears Lower Heater)

Bl28 (regulates
Lower Heater and
Bladder function
Bl32 (regulates
Lower Heater.
'Experience' pt.)

**Stagnation of Qi**

Sp9 (moves Sp Qi)

Sp7 ('Experience' pt
for Dysuria)

Li3 (regulates
circulation of Qi)

Bl28 (disperses Qi
of Lower Heater)

Bl32 (moves Qi at
Lower Heater.
'Experience'pt.)

flushed complexion with a feeling of heaviness in the head and vertigo, whilst there is frequently a bitter taste in the mouth. The patient may be either constipated, or have difficult (obstructed) watery stools. The pulse is rapid, the tongue reddish with a thin yellow or greasy white coat.

Points to remove the heat and damp are used, such as Li2 (Xingjian), Ki9 (Fuliu), Sp9 (Yinlingquan), Bl28 (Pangguangshu) and Bl32 (Ciliao).

## (d) Stagnation of Qi

This starts with acute pain and swelling in the lower abdomen almost from the date of conception, accompanied by dysuria, and lasts through until almost the last month of gestation. There is congestion in the chest and heartburn, the patient is often depressed and experiences discomfort when lying stretched straight out. The pulse is deep and wiry, the tongue swollen with tooth-marks and a thin sticky coat.

To move the Qi, we could use Sp9 (Yinlingquan), Li3 (Taichong), Sp7 (Ligou), Bl28 (Pangguangshu) and Bl32 (Ciliao).

(The points recommended in this section are selected from Zhang Ting-Liang's translation of the Zhong Yi Fu Ke Shou Ce, from the Zhejiang College. There are, of course, others which can be used at the practitioner's discretion, but these do seem to be extremely appropriate for their purpose.)

# ABORTION AND MISCARRIAGE

Abortion is the evacuation of an uncompletely developed foetus of less than three months old, or before sixteen weeks. Miscarriage is discharge of the foetus before twenty-eight weeks when, according to current law, the foetus is viable. A baby born alive after twenty-eight weeks is called premature, and if born dead during this period is called a stillbirth.

There are many causes of abortion, and the majority occur within the first three months of pregnancy, often at the time when menstruation would normally take place.

Early separation of the ovum from the uterine wall can have several causes, such as resulting from a fall, the use of certain drugs or aperients by the mother, diseases of the mother (e.g. nephritis, untreated diabetes, specific fevers) or the presence of fibroids, tumours, or a prolapsed or retroverted uterus. Incompetence of the cervical internal os, either congenital or acquired, is a factor to be considered, as this acts as the sphincter of the uterus.

Endocrine causes are very common, more notably a deficiency of progesterone, whilst a deficiency of folic acid may ocasionally be responsible.

Congenital malformation of the embryo is a frequent cause, as is hydatidiform degeneration of the chorion and faulty implantation, whilst emotional stress is an extremely important cause which must not be overlooked.

Abortions are divided into two types – *threatened* and *inevitable*.

## Threatened abortion

This takes place at the end of the second or third month of pregnancy, the main symptom being slight haemorrhage (although occasionally severe) but little pain apart from slight backache and (rarely) some painful contractions. The presence of the usual preceding signs of pregnancy – amenorrhoea, morning sickness, frequency, and enlargement of the breasts, serves to distinguish it from dysfunctional uterine bleeding. The presence of the embryo can be confirmed by examination by ultrasound and blood or urine tests for the presence of chorionic gonadotrophins.

Treatment is usually by bed rest for at least a week, followed by a few days a month late when the next period is due. A sedative may also be prescribed.

## Inevitable abortion

This means that there is no hope of saving the pregnancy, as the whole of the ovum has become detached. The chief signs are pain and haemorrhaging, and on examination the internal os will be found to be dilated. If the abortion is *complete* the whole of the contents are expelled – foetus, placenta and chorion. If it is *incomplete* some or all of the chorionic tissue may be left behind, and will have to be evacuated in theatre.

The first thing to make very clear is that on no account is acupuncture for these conditions to be given *during* pregnancy. They are to be used as a preventative measure to be taken when the patient presents with a desire for a successful pregnancy but with a history of previous miscarriages or abortions. The treatments will therefore form part of an overall assessment of the patient's physical and mental/emotional condition, but certain specific patterns have been described in the literature.

The more usual syndromes are:
(a) Blood deficiency ⎫ often described
(b) Qi deficiency ⎭ together as deficiency of Qi and blood.
(c) Kidney Qi deficiency
(d) Stagnation of liver Qi
(e) Heat in the blood
(f) Dysfunction of Chong Mai and Ren Mai channels

## (a) Blood deficiency
Apart from the vaginal bleeding during pregnancy there will be some abdominal distension and often a feeling as if 'things were falling down' in the lower abdomen. There is usually some low back ache, the complexion will be yellowish, and there will be a tendency for dizziness, palpitations, and insomnia. The pulse will be fine and weak and the tongue pale.

## (b) Qi deficiency
This will present with frequent bleeding at an early stage in the pregnancy, with the discharge of a watery, yellowish fluid rather than blood. As with blood deficiency, there may be abdominal distension with the same 'falling down' sensation internally, with soreness in the loins. The complexion will be paler, whiter, with a heavy sensation in the head accompanied by a tendency to vertigo. Above all is a general weakness and lassitude, with anorexia and a lack of taste. The pulse will be weak and sliding, the tongue will have a thin white coat.

Where Qi and Blood deficiency are combined, the general lassitude and weakness will be increased and, as there will almost invariably be a basic kidney deficiency, there will often be the passage of frequent clear urine and a clear, watery leucorrhoea.

Treatment will depend upon which of the deficiencies is the most prominent, but it is suggested to select from the following points:

CV4 (Guanyuan), CV6 (Qihai), Sp6 (Sanyinjiao), St36 (Zusanli), Bl17 (Geshu), Bl20 (Pishu) and Bl23 (Shenshu).

## (c) Deficiency of Kidney Qi
As the kidneys are involved the tendency to pain in the lumbar area will be prominent, whilst there will be weakness in the limbs accompanied by vertigo and a tendency to tinnitus. Sleep will be poor and there will be frequency of urination with a long, clear, copious stream. The pulse will be weak (especially in the Chi or Kidney position), the tongue pale.

To tonify the kidneys, Bl23 (Shenshu) and Bl28 (Pangguanshu) are recommended, with moxa to CV4 (Guanyuan) and GV4 (Mingmen). As a general stimulant one could add St36 (Zusanli).

## (d) Stagnation of Liver Qi
The foetal movements will be noticeable, possibly accompanied by abdominal pain. There may be lack of appetite or a vomiting of sour, acid water, congestion in the chest and belching, with pain in the ribs. The pulse is wiry and slippery, the tongue has a thick greasy coat.

Disperse the congestion: Bl15 (Xinshu), Bl18 (Ganshu), Bl20 (Pishu), Li2 (Xingjian), TH3 (Zhongzhu) or TH6 (Zhigou), CV4 (Guanyuan).

## (e) Heat in the Blood
Typically there will be a loss of light to bright red blood. The patient will have a flushed complexion and will be irritable. There will be dryness in the mouth, with thirst; the urine will be yellowish and scanty, the faeces dry, giving rise to constipation. The pulse will be rapid and either fine and slippery or large and empty; the tongue red with a dry yellow fur.

Clear the heat with Bl15 (Xinshu), Bl18 (Ganshu), Bl20 (Pinshu), Sp10 (Xuehai), Sp9 (Yinlingquan), and CV3 (Zhongji).

## (f) Dysfunction of Chong Mai and Ren Mai
Previous histories of miscarriages would have included heavy blood loss with fainting spells or, in serious cases, a continuous seepage of blood. The patient would feel generally weak,

# ABORTION AND MISCARRIAGE

## Deficiency of Qi and Blood

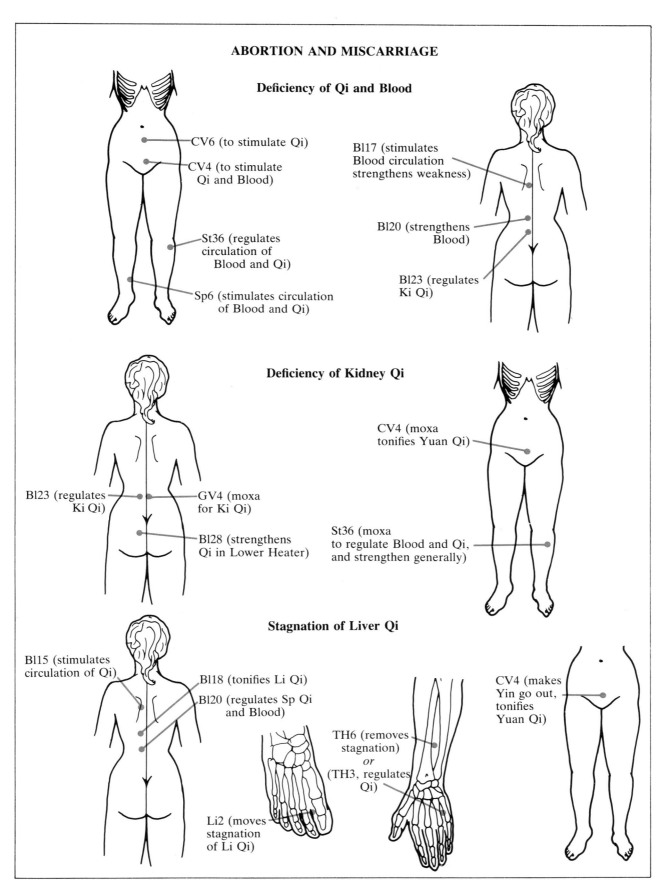

CV6 (to stimulate Qi)

CV4 (to stimulate Qi and Blood)

St36 (regulates circulation of Blood and Qi)

Sp6 (stimulates circulation of Blood and Qi)

Bl17 (stimulates Blood circulation strengthens weakness)

Bl20 (strengthens Blood)

Bl23 (regulates Ki Qi)

## Deficiency of Kidney Qi

Bl23 (regulates Ki Qi)

GV4 (moxa for Ki Qi)

Bl28 (strengthens Qi in Lower Heater)

CV4 (moxa tonifies Yuan Qi)

St36 (moxa to regulate Blood and Qi, and strengthen generally)

## Stagnation of Liver Qi

Bl15 (stimulates circulation of Qi)

Bl18 (tonifies Li Qi)

Bl20 (regulates Sp Qi and Blood)

Li2 (moves stagnation of Li Qi)

TH6 (removes stagnation)
*or*
(TH3, regulates Qi)

CV4 (makes Yin go out, tonifies Yuan Qi)

**Heat in Blood**

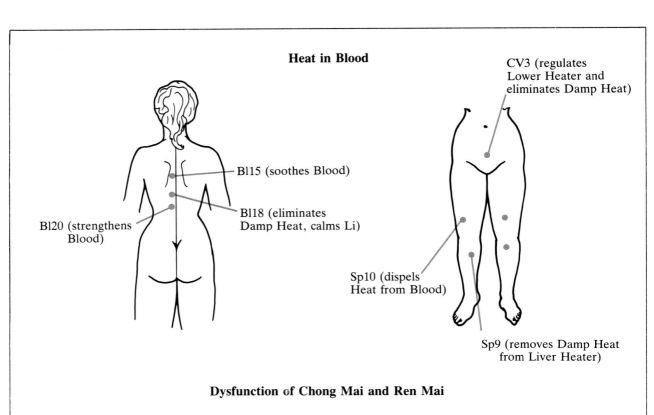

Bl15 (soothes Blood)

Bl18 (eliminates
Damp Heat, calms Li)

Bl20 (strengthens
Blood)

CV3 (regulates
Lower Heater and
eliminates Damp Heat)

Sp10 (dispels
Heat from Blood)

Sp9 (removes Damp Heat
from Liver Heater)

**Dysfunction of Chong Mai and Ren Mai**

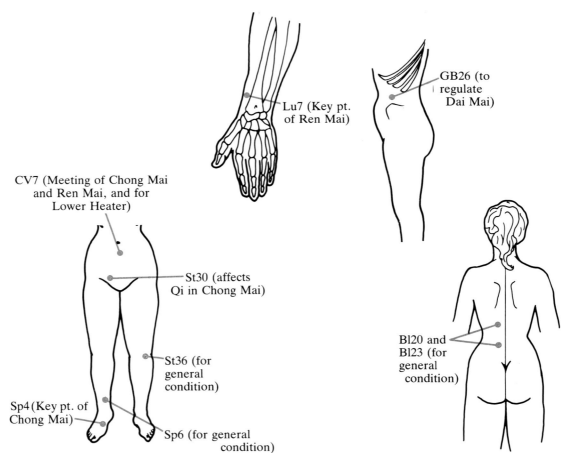

Lu7 (Key pt.
of Ren Mai)

GB26 (to
regulate
Dai Mai)

CV7 (Meeting of Chong Mai
and Ren Mai, and for
Lower Heater)

St30 (affects
Qi in Chong Mai)

St36 (for
general
condition)

Sp4 (Key pt. of
Chong Mai)

Sp6 (for general
condition)

Bl20 and
Bl23 (for
general
condition)

particularly in the legs and low back, and abdominal pain would be relieved by pressure. The pulse would be weak, the tongue pale with a light coat.

We would have to use the command points of the Irregular vessels concerned – Sp4 (Gongsun) and Lu7 (Lieque); also suggested would be St30 (Qichong), CV7 (Yinjiao) – the meeting point of Chong Mai and Ren Mai and also to affect the Lower Heater; CV4 (Guanyuan), and possibly GB26 (Daimai) to regulate Dai Mai. Sp6 (Sanyinjiao) and St36 (Zusanli), Bl20 (Pishu) and Bl23 (Shenshu) may be used for the general condition.

The practitioner will notice that as these treatments are to be given as a preventative measure and therefore used before pregnancy is achieved, the use of points otherwise prohibited is quite satisfactory.

# THE INDUCTION OF LABOUR

One aspect of acupuncture which has particularly caught the public's imagination during recent years is its application for pain during childbirth. Many Chinese practitioners to whom I have spoken tend to regard childbirth as a natural function, to be interfered with as little as possible, and feel that acupuncture should be used mainly when there is a weakness in the uterine contractions, when its application can be regarded as assisting nature rather than interfering with its function. To the best of my knowledge acupuncture in this respect has not been used to any great extent in the Western world, but Dr Wilfred Pererra of Sri Lanka has presided over several thousand cases with extremely impressive results.

Normal childbirth may be divided into three stages:

1) From the onset of labour pains to full dilation of the cervix – usually about 15 hours for a primigravida and 8 hours for a multipara.
2) From full dilatation to actual delivery – usually one to two hours.
3) From delivery until one hour after the expulsion of the placenta.

In the case of malposition of the foetus, a well-known treatment is the use of moxa on Bl67 (Zhiyen) for twenty minutes every day for four to five days. The patient is usually presented with a moxa-roll or green-stick moxa and instructed in how to perform this for herself. This works particularly well in cases of breech presentation, when the patient will frequently report feeling the baby turn itself into the correct position. It is most effective if used before the 34th week of pregnancy. Another technique, to raise the placenta and the foetus, is moxa (on salt) to CV8 (Shenque).

To stimulate labour, the basic formula given by most Chinese sources is Bl31 (Shangliao), Bl32 (Ciliao), Co4 (Hegu) and Sp6 (Sanyinjiao), either needle manipulation for fifteen to thirty minutes or electrical stimulation, but alternative combinations have been tried, such as Co4 (Hegu), Sp6 (Sanyinjiao), GB21 (Jianjing) and Bl67 (Zhiyen), or Co4 (Hegu), Sp6 (Sanyinjiao), GV1 (Changqiang) and Sp9 (Yinlingquan).

The object of all these points is to regulate the Qi, move the blood, and strengthen the contractions.

To stimulate the induction, tonification of Co4 (Hegu), Sp6 (Sanyinjiao), Bl32 (Ciliao), CV4 (Guanyuan) and St36 (Zusanli) is recommended, or possibly Co4 (Hegu), Sp6 (Sanyinjiao), Bl31 (Shangliao) and Li3 (Taichong). As an 'experience' point, the use of Bl32 (Ciliao) seems preferable to Bl31 (Shangliao).

When there are weak contractions and the cervix is slow to dilate, stimulate either Co4 (Hegu) and St36 (Zusanli) or Co4 (Hegu) and Sp6 (Sanyinjiao), whilst for an atonic uterus tonify St30 (Qichong), GB34 (Yanglingquan), CV3 (Zhongji) and then sedate Sp6 (Sanyinjiao).

# INDUCTION OF LABOUR

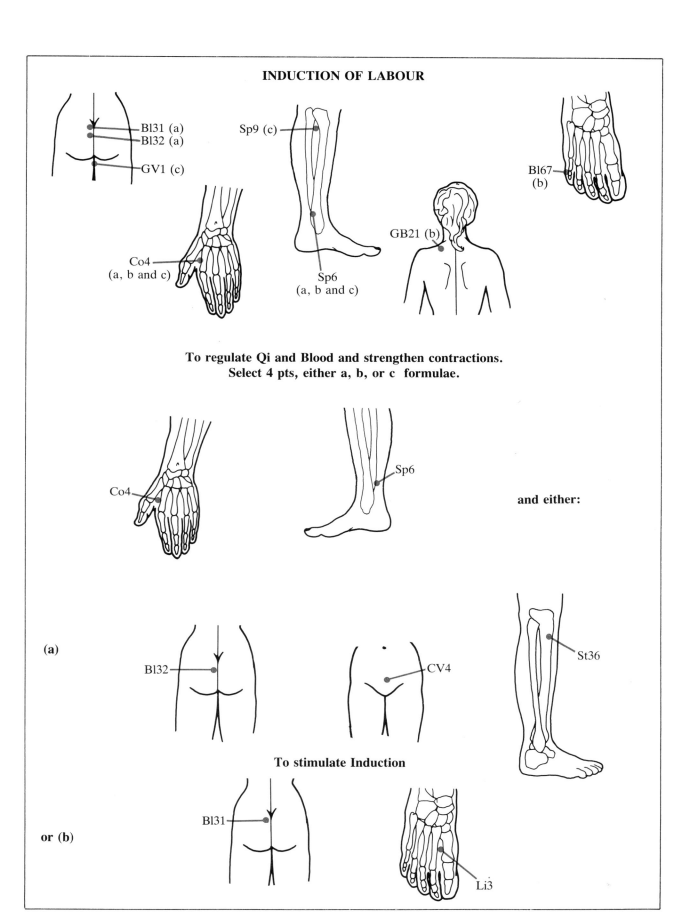

Bl31 (a)
Bl32 (a)
GV1 (c)
Sp9 (c)
Bl67 (b)
Co4 (a, b and c)
Sp6 (a, b and c)
GB21 (b)

**To regulate Qi and Blood and strengthen contractions.
Select 4 pts, either a, b, or c formulae.**

Co4

Sp6

**and either:**

**(a)**

Bl32

CV4

St36

**To stimulate Induction**

**or (b)**

Bl31

Li3

99

**Weak Contractions**

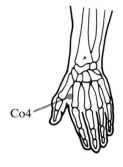

Co4

**and either:**

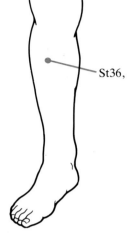

St36,

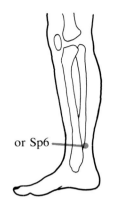

or Sp6

**Atonic Uterus**

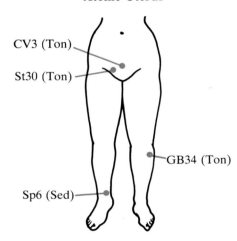

CV3 (Ton)

St30 (Ton)

GB34 (Ton)

Sp6 (Sed)

**Pain during Labour**

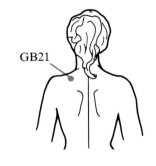

GB21

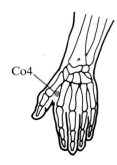

Co4

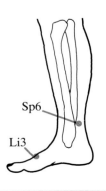

Sp6

Li3

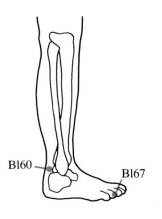

Bl60

Bl67

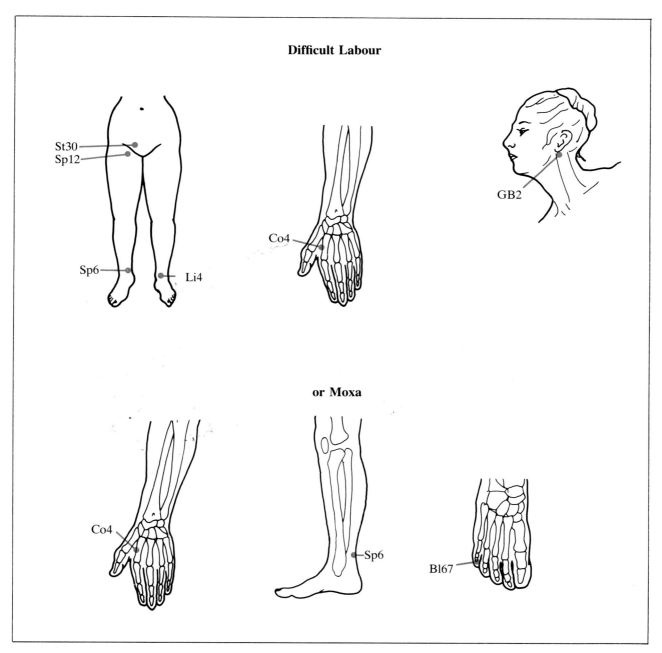

**Difficult Labour**

**or Moxa**

Pain during labour may be treated by either GB21 (Jianjing), Co4 (Hegu), Sp6 (Sanyinjiao), Li3 (Taichong), Bl60 (Kunlun) and Bl67 (Zhiyen) or Co4 (Hegu), Sp6 (Sanyinjiao), Li3 (Taichong), Bl60 (Kunlun) and CV4 (Guanyuan). Strong pressure on Bl60 (Kunlun) may also help.

In cases of difficult labour, stimulate Sp12 (Chongmen), Li4 (Zhongfen), St30 (Qichong), Co4 (Hegu), Sp6 (Sanyinjiao) and GB2 (Tinghui), or moxa Co4 (Hegu) and Sp6 (Sanyinjiao) and burn three cones on Bl67 (Zhiyin).

Ear points may also be used in conjunction with the body points, usually Uterus and Endocrine, with the needles being inserted and stimulated every five minutes for about twenty minutes.

Dr Pererra's own treatment, as given at a talk he gave at a British Acupuncture Association Congress, was firstly a sedative needle in GV20 (Baihui) to relax the patient, and then needles inserted into Co4 (Hegu) bilaterally and into Sp6 (Sanyinjiao) on the opposite side to the doctor.

During the first stage, electro-stimulation was applied to the leg points (Sp6) only, using either a dense/disperse or an interrupted current.

During the second stage, strong manual stimulation was given to Co4 (Hegu).

During the third stage, moxa was applied to Bl60 (Kunlun).

As noted earlier, Dr Pererra attended several thousand cases with marked success, and during his talk he made several pertinent observations, including:

1) Acupuncture should be used in conjunction with the usual routine measures taken for the normal delivery.

2) Acupuncture gives a pain-free delivery.

3) The stress and effort placed upon the mother is considerably less.

4) There is far less chance of post-partum haemorrhage.

5) Due to the great decrease in time taken when acupuncture is used, there is far less chance of injury to the foetal head, leading to an increase in the mental development of babies delivered by this means.

6) There was an almost 100 per cent absence of ophthalmia neonatorum.

# Part Three:
# Post-partum disorders

# RETENTION OF THE PLACENTA

A condition more usually due to weakness of the mother after the delivery, it may also be due to a general weakness of Qi and 'stagnation of blood' in the uterus. In both cases we must encourage the Qi and move the blood in the pelvic basin. The usual points recommended are CV3 (Zhongji), Co4 (Hegu), Sp6 (Sanyin-jiao), GB21 (Jiangjing) and Bl60 (Kunlun), but points such as CV4 (Guanyuan) or CV6 (Qihai), Sp8 (Diji) and St31 (Biguan) may also be considered. The key points of the Yinqiao and the Yinwei (Ki6 Zhaohai and Lu7 Lieque) have also been used.

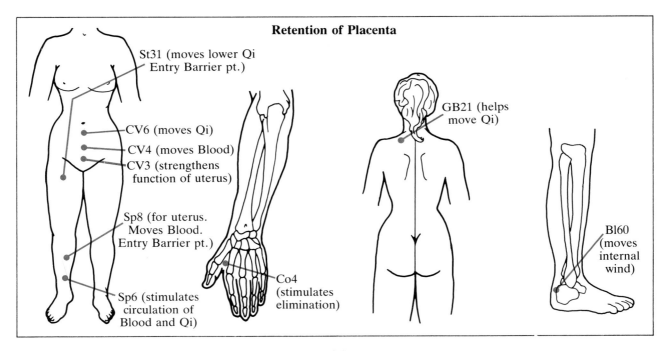

**Retention of Placenta**

St31 (moves lower Qi Entry Barrier pt.)

CV6 (moves Qi)

CV4 (moves Blood)

CV3 (strengthens function of uterus)

Sp8 (for uterus. Moves Blood. Entry Barrier pt.)

Sp6 (stimulates circulation of Blood and Qi)

Co4 (stimulates elimination)

GB21 (helps move Qi)

Bl60 (moves internal wind)

# RETENTION OF LOCHIA

Lochia is the term used to denote the residual bleeding which takes place after labour. It is normally inoffensive and bright red for a few days, after which it becomes brown and more scanty as healing of the uterine wall occurs. It normally stops after eight or ten days.

Retention of the lochia means that there is a failure to discharge this residual blood and amniotic fluid – the lochia is persistent and offensive and usually indicates that some part of the placenta or membranes has been left behind in the uterus during the third stage of labour – this frequently becomes septic, giving rise to the offensive smell.

The reason for the failure to discharge the lochia completely is usually put down to weakness – due possibly to undue haemorrhage during the delivery, or to a general weakness in the patient, resulting in a general weakness of blood and Qi or to a stagnation.

General exhaustion would present signs of a pale, sallow complexion, vertigo, tinnitus, general fatigue, and a light scanty discharge. The abdomen would feel soft and atonic with no real pain but an empty, distended feeling, better for pressure. The pulse would be fine and weak, the tongue pale with little or no fur.

Treatment would call for general stimulation of such points as CV4 (Guanyuan) and CV6 (Qihai), Bl17 (Geshu), Bl20 (Pishu), and Bl23 (Shenshu), Sp6 (Sanyinjiao) and St36 (Zusanli).

If the cause is a congestion of Qi, which fails to move the blood, the abdomen will be distended but there will be pain radiating to the lumbar area and the hips. The pulse will be more wiry and the tongue light red.

Points to regulate the Qi should be used, such as CV6 (Qihai), St25 (Tianshu), St36 (Zusanli) and Bl22 (Sanjiaoshu). St37 (Pohu) will help the Qi to descend.

Stagnation of blood is an altogether more serious condition, and calls for immediate treatment. There will be either a scanty discharge or even a complete suppression. There may be vomiting and dyspepsia, whilst the lower abdomen will be acutely painful (worse on pressure) with distension and fixed lumps. The pulse will be deep and slow, the tongue slightly purple or with purple markings.

To activate the blood, typical points could be CV4 (Guanyuan), St29 (Guilai), Sp6 (Sanyinjiao), Sp10 (Xuehai), Li3 (Taichong) and Bl32 (Ciliao) – all naturally in tonification.

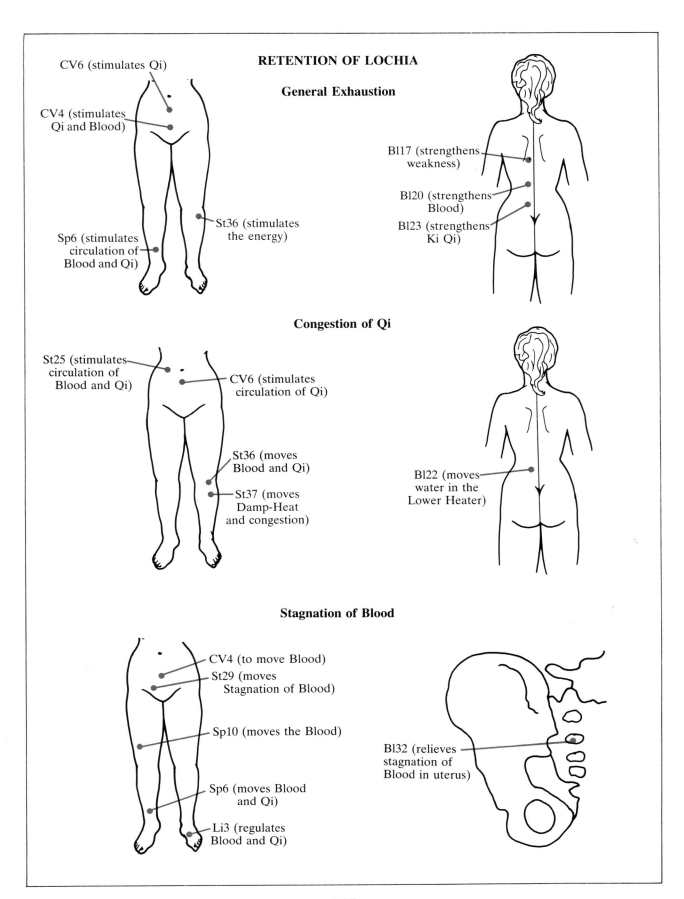

**RETENTION OF LOCHIA**

**General Exhaustion**

CV6 (stimulates Qi)

CV4 (stimulates Qi and Blood)

Sp6 (stimulates circulation of Blood and Qi)

St36 (stimulates the energy)

Bl17 (strengthens weakness)

Bl20 (strengthens Blood)

Bl23 (strengthens Ki Qi)

**Congestion of Qi**

St25 (stimulates circulation of Blood and Qi)

CV6 (stimulates circulation of Qi)

St36 (moves Blood and Qi)

St37 (moves Damp-Heat and congestion)

Bl22 (moves water in the Lower Heater)

**Stagnation of Blood**

CV4 (to move Blood)

St29 (moves Stagnation of Blood)

Sp10 (moves the Blood)

Sp6 (moves Blood and Qi)

Li3 (regulates Blood and Qi)

Bl32 (relieves stagnation of Blood in uterus)

# LOCHIORRHOEA

This is the exact opposite of the previous condition, and is usually considered to be present once the lochia have continued for over three weeks after delivery.

The three main causes are, according to TCM, Weakness of Qi, 'Hot Blood in the Liver Channel', and Blood Stagnation.

## Weakness of Qi
This is ascribed to a deficiency of Ren Mai and Chong Mai brought on by haemorrhage during delivery, and presents as a continuous thin, slightly yellow lochia accompanied by pallor, weakness, palpitations, vertigo, dyspnoea, lack of appetite, and a soft swollen abdomen with an aversion to cold. The pulse is weak and hollow and the tongue is pale with little fur.

To tonify the Qi and constrict the blood vessels, one could use CV4 (Guanyuan), CV6 (Qihai), Sp6 (Sanyinjiao), Ki3 (Taixi), Bl20 (Pishu), Bl23 (Shenshu) and St36 (Zusanli).

## 'Hot Blood in the Liver Channel'
This causes the blood to flow outside its normal channels, and results in an unchecked flow of bright red, offensive blood accompanied by heartburn, thirst, and a reddish complexion. The pulse is thready and rapid and the tongue red with light yellowish fur.

This is the usual picture of a relative excess of Yang due to a deficient Yin, so we must fortify the Yin and disperse the heat: CV6 (Qihai), CV3 (Zhongji), Sp6 (Sanyinjiao), Sp10 (Xuehai), Li2 (Xingjian) and Li8 (Ququan) are suggested by most sources.

## Blood Stagnation
This will naturally give a dark, purplish lochia containing clots, having a repulsive smell. The lower abdomen will be painful and (as in retention of lochia) will have lumps worse with pressure. In severe cases there may be fever and constipation, with possible delirium and a dark grey complexion. The pulse is usually hesitant, deep and wiry, and the tongue purplish.

To move the stagnation, CV4 (Guanyuan), St29 (Guilai), Sp6 (Sanyinjiao), Sp10 (Xuehai), Li3 (Taichong) and Bl32 (Ciliao) could be used (as for the stagnation causing retention).

# LOCHIORRHOEA

## Weakness of Qi

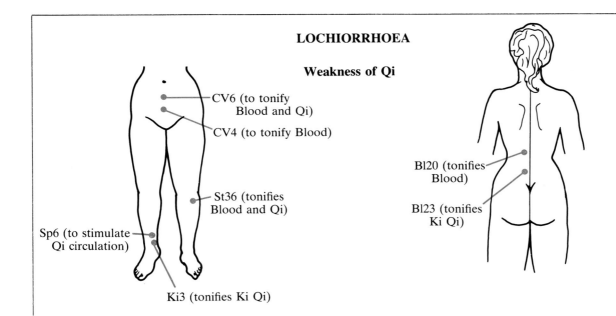

CV6 (to tonify Blood and Qi)

CV4 (to tonify Blood)

St36 (tonifies Blood and Qi)

Sp6 (to stimulate Qi circulation)

Ki3 (tonifies Ki Qi)

Bl20 (tonifies Blood)

Bl23 (tonifies Ki Qi)

## Hot Blood in Liver Channel

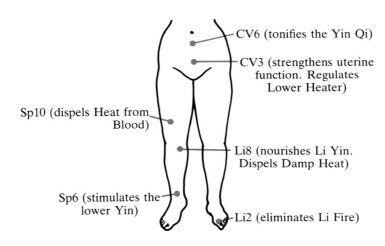

CV6 (tonifies the Yin Qi)

CV3 (strengthens uterine function. Regulates Lower Heater)

Sp10 (dispels Heat from Blood)

Li8 (nourishes Li Yin. Dispels Damp Heat)

Sp6 (stimulates the lower Yin)

Li2 (eliminates Li Fire)

## Blood Stagnation

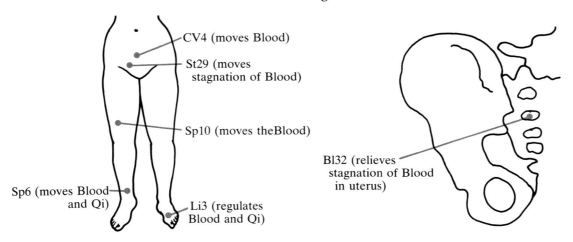

CV4 (moves Blood)

St29 (moves stagnation of Blood)

Sp10 (moves theBlood)

Sp6 (moves Blood and Qi)

Li3 (regulates Blood and Qi)

Bl32 (relieves stagnation of Blood in uterus)

# ABDOMINAL PAIN

Continuous abdominal pain after delivery is, traditionally, due to either a stagnation of blood, deficiency of blood, or a 'deficiency cold'.

## Stagnation of Blood

This is usually a concomitant of 'Retention of Lochia' and presents with similar symptoms and the use of the same points: Co4 (Hegu), St29 (Guilai), Sp6 (Sanyinjiao), Sp10 (Xuehai), Li3 (Taichong) and Bl32 (Ciliao).

## Deficiency of Blood

This is brought on by haemorrhage during delivery. The picture is slightly different from that of retention of lochia due to blood and Qi deficiency, in that there is a general mild continuous ache, better for pressure and warmth. There will be the usual general malaise, possibly with vertigo and/or tinnitus, and a possible mild fever with sweating at night. The pulse is thready and slow, the tongue pale with a thin white coat.

To nourish the blood, stimulate points such as CV4 (Guanyuan), CV6 (Qihai), St36 (Zusanli), Sp6 (Sanyinjiao), Bl17 (Geshu), Bl20 (Pishu) and Bl23 (Shenshu).

## Deficiency Cold

This occurs when there is an invasion of cold to the uterus in a patient already weakened by loss of blood during the delivery. The lower abdominal pain will radiate to the umbilicus and be better for warmth and pressure, the lochia will be scanty, and complexion pale, the limbs will feel cold, and the patient will generally lack energy. The pulse will be deep, weak and retarded, the tongue pale with a thin white coating.

We must naturally warm the channels, but also it will be necessary to stimulate the replenishment of the lost blood, possibly by moxa on CV4 (Guanyuan), CV12 (Zhongwan), St25 (Tianshu), St36 (Zusanli), Sp6 (Sanyinjiao), and Li3 (Taichong).

# ABDOMINAL PAIN

## Stagnation of Blood

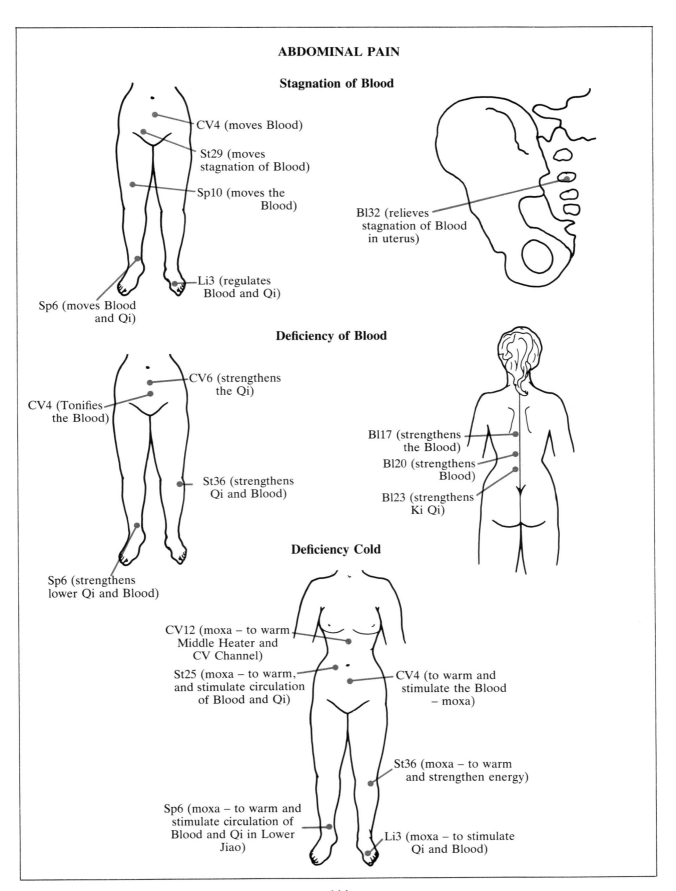

CV4 (moves Blood)

St29 (moves stagnation of Blood)

Sp10 (moves the Blood)

Bl32 (relieves stagnation of Blood in uterus)

Li3 (regulates Blood and Qi)

Sp6 (moves Blood and Qi)

## Deficiency of Blood

CV6 (strengthens the Qi)

CV4 (Tonifies the Blood)

St36 (strengthens Qi and Blood)

Bl17 (strengthens the Blood)

Bl20 (strengthens Blood)

Bl23 (strengthens Ki Qi)

Sp6 (strengthens lower Qi and Blood)

## Deficiency Cold

CV12 (moxa – to warm Middle Heater and CV Channel)

St25 (moxa – to warm, and stimulate circulation of Blood and Qi)

CV4 (to warm and stimulate the Blood – moxa)

St36 (moxa – to warm and strengthen energy)

Sp6 (moxa – to warm and stimulate circulation of Blood and Qi in Lower Jiao)

Li3 (moxa – to stimulate Qi and Blood)

# FAINTING AFTER DELIVERY

This can be an alarming occurrence, and is regarded in the ancient writings as being due to an upward reflux of ecchymotic blood in the liver channel. It is thought to have three possible causes:

## (a) Deficiency of Qi
This is possibly the most likely one, and is due to the general strain of delivery and a poor constitution. This will give a sudden syncope with pallor, icy coldness in the limbs, sweating on the forehead, and a weak and thready pulse with a pale tongue.

Tonify the Qi with CV3 (Zhongji), CV4 (Guanyuan), CV12 (Zhongwan), St36 (Zusanli), St 25 (Tianshu), Bl20 (Pishu), Bl22 (Sanjiaoshu). GV26 (Renzhong) may also be considered.

## (b) Deficiency of Blood
This is brought on by haemorrhaging during delivery. The patient will again present pallor and an outbreak of sweat on the forehead.

There may be palpitations and nausea, with a suffocating feeling. The pulse will be hollow and weak, the tongue pale.

Tonify the blood via Bl17 (Geshu), Bl20 (Pishu), Bl23 (Shenshu), Bl38 (Gaohuangshu), St36 (Zusanli), Sp6 (Sanyinjiao) and Ki3 (Taixi).

## (c) Blood Stagnation
Fainting due to this is extremely serious. As was mentioned in the treatment of retention of lochia, it is an 'emergency situation'. The patient will exhibit panting and loss of breath, the complexion will turn purple, the hands will be tightly clenched and there will be a desire to vomit. Apart from the actual syncopic episode there will be a distended pain in the lower abdomen made worse by pressure. The pulse is deep and hesitant, the tongue purplish.

The usual points for stagnation of blood are used: CV4 (Guanyuan), St29 (Guilai), Sp6 (Sanyinjiao), Sp10 (Xuehai), Li3 (Taichong) and Bl32 (Ciliao).

# FAINTING AFTER DELIVERY

## Deficiency of Qi

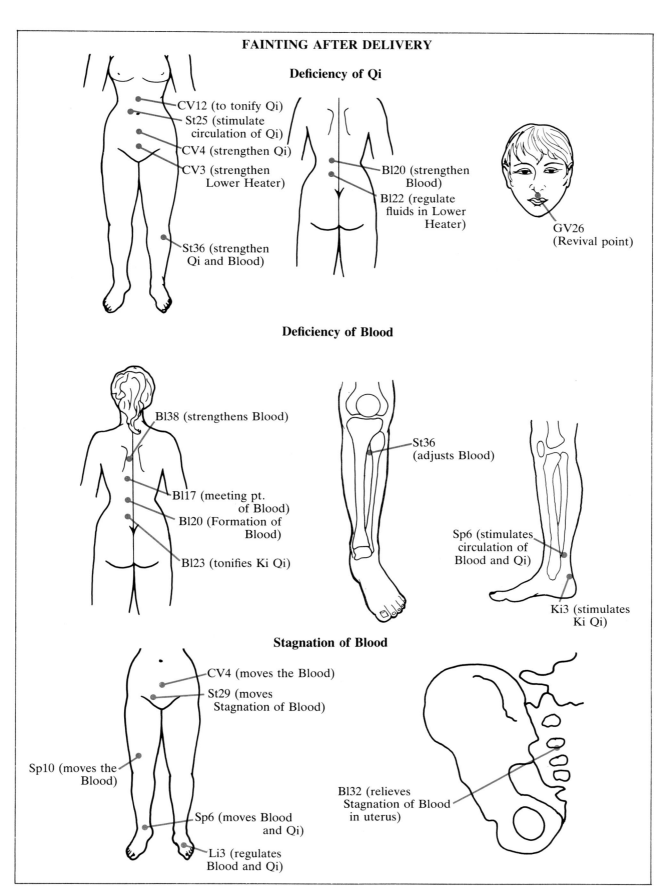

CV12 (to tonify Qi)

St25 (stimulate circulation of Qi)

CV4 (strengthen Qi)

CV3 (strengthen Lower Heater)

St36 (strengthen Qi and Blood)

Bl20 (strengthen Blood)

Bl22 (regulate fluids in Lower Heater)

GV26 (Revival point)

## Deficiency of Blood

Bl38 (strengthens Blood)

Bl17 (meeting pt. of Blood)

Bl20 (Formation of Blood)

Bl23 (tonifies Ki Qi)

St36 (adjusts Blood)

Sp6 (stimulates circulation of Blood and Qi)

Ki3 (stimulates Ki Qi)

## Stagnation of Blood

CV4 (moves the Blood)

St29 (moves Stagnation of Blood)

Sp10 (moves the Blood)

Sp6 (moves Blood and Qi)

Li3 (regulates Blood and Qi)

Bl32 (relieves Stagnation of Blood in uterus)

113

# FEVER

The causes of post-partum fever are as numerous as the causes of fever under any other circumstances, and although the literature lists them as 'post-partum fevers' they would have occurred whether the patient was 'post-partum' or not. The only factor is that the strain of delivery has most likely so depleted the patient that her body's defences are in a weakened condition, which renders her more susceptible to infection of any sort.

The only really specific one is that due to *Obstructed Lactation*. In this case there will be a discharge of lochia with the fever, coming on two to three days after delivery. The breasts will be swollen with palpable lumps and, as the name implies, there will be difficulty over the lactation. The pulse will be rapid and wiry and the tongue pale. Treatment will be directed to removing the obstruction and will employ several local points which have both a local and a general 'de-obstructing' effect – suggested are St18 (Rugan), Li14 (Qimen), CV17 (Shanzhong), P7 (Daling), St40 (Fenglong) and Li2 (Xingjian).

As we have seen, in a weakened condition the patient will more readily fall prey to external inimical influences, and fever due to *External Pathogenic Factors* would present with emaciation and listlessness, a sallow complexion, dislike of the cold, headache and dizziness. She will usually complain of general aches, particularly in the lumbar area, and the fever will *not* be accompanied by sweating. The pulse will be superficial and thready, the tongue pale with a thin white coat.

Treatment will consist of stimulating the blood and endeavouring to encourage perspiration – GB20 (Fengchi), St36 (Zusanli), Lu7 (Lieque), Co4 (Hegu), Bl12 (Fengmen), Bl20 (Pishu) and Bl23 (Shenshu) will help.

Specifically to produce sweating, reduce Co4 (Hegu) and tonify Ki7 (Fuliu) or (the treatment of the Su Wen) reduce Lu9 (Taiyuan) and Lu10 (Yuji) and tonify Sp1 (Yinbai) and Sp2 (Dadu).

What is sometimes called 'False Fever' is a condition of *Yin Xu with Internal Heat*. In this condition the fever is worse in the afternoon and, in distinction from the previous case, there is no aversion to cold. There will also be night sweats, there is a malar flush, and sometimes the palms and soles feel hot. Because of the internal heat there will be thirst, with a preference for cold drinks, but the patient will not drink much. There will be dry stools and a concentrated urine. The pulse is rapid and thready, the tongue red and dry.

Points to clear the heat could include Co11 (Quchi), Ki6 (Zhaohai), Sp10 (Xuehai), TH3 (Zhongzhu) and Ki3 (Taixi). Points to tonify the Yin would be the usual ones such as Ki3 (Taixi), CV6 (Qihai), Ki7 (Fuliu) etc.

Sometimes a fever may be due to nothing more esoteric than *indigestion* (which TCM describes as 'Fever due to Food Injury'!). Here, the principle symptoms will be acid regurgitation and belching, abdominal pain and swelling

# FEVER

## Obstructed Lactation

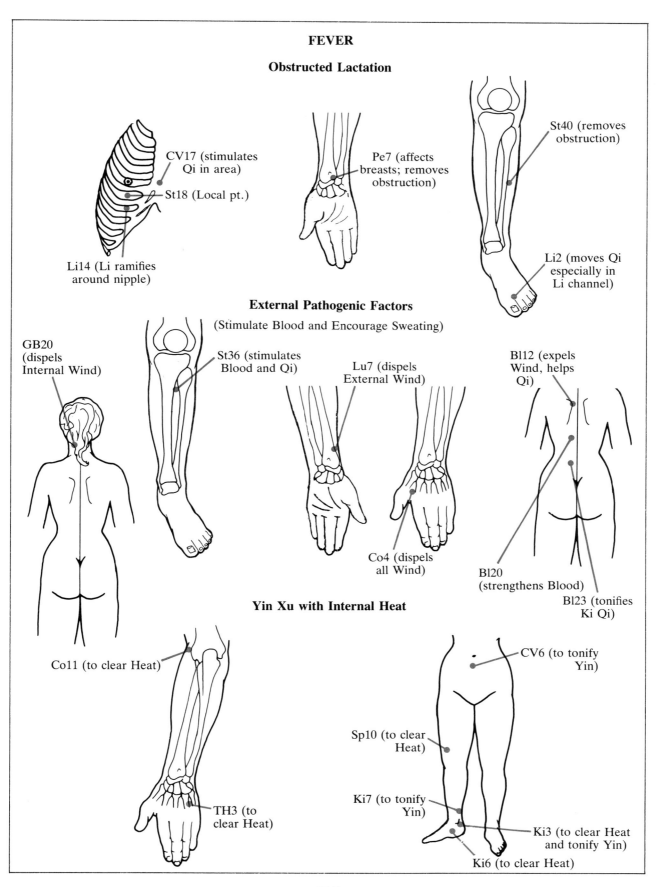

CV17 (stimulates Qi in area)

St18 (Local pt.)

Li14 (Li ramifies around nipple)

Pe7 (affects breasts; removes obstruction)

St40 (removes obstruction)

Li2 (moves Qi especially in Li channel)

## External Pathogenic Factors

### (Stimulate Blood and Encourage Sweating)

GB20 (dispels Internal Wind)

St36 (stimulates Blood and Qi)

Lu7 (dispels External Wind)

Bl12 (expels Wind, helps Qi)

Co4 (dispels all Wind)

Bl20 (strengthens Blood)

Bl23 (tonifies Ki Qi)

## Yin Xu with Internal Heat

Co11 (to clear Heat)

TH3 (to clear Heat)

CV6 (to tonify Yin)

Sp10 (to clear Heat)

Ki7 (to tonify Yin)

Ki3 (to clear Heat and tonify Yin)

Ki6 (to clear Heat)

115

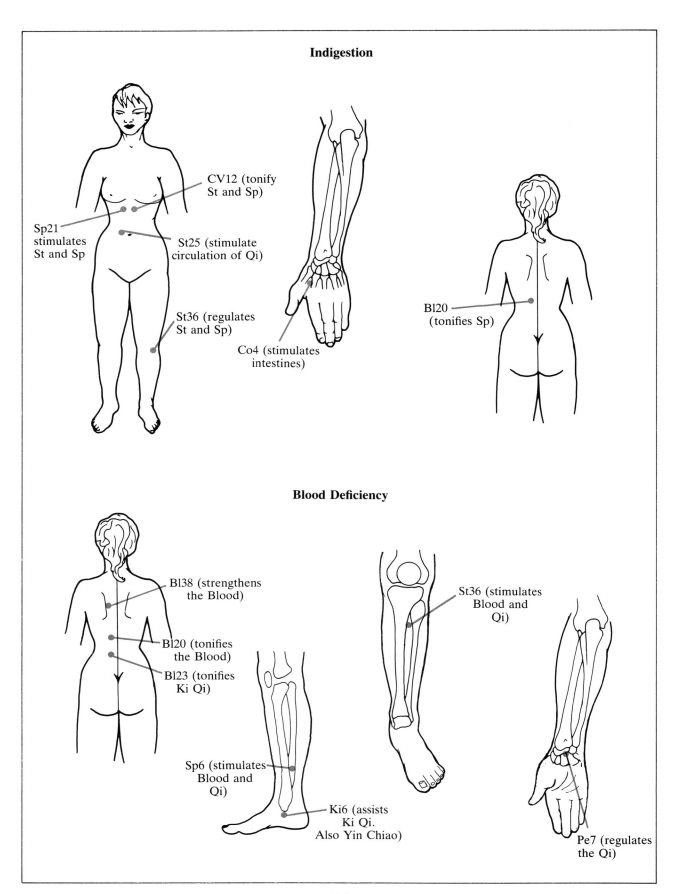

**Indigestion**

CV12 (tonify
St and Sp)

Sp21
stimulates
St and Sp

St25 (stimulate
circulation of Qi)

St36 (regulates
St and Sp)

Co4 (stimulates
intestines)

Bl20
(tonifies Sp)

**Blood Deficiency**

Bl38 (strengthens
the Blood)

Bl20 (tonifies
the Blood)

Bl23 (tonifies
Ki Qi)

St36 (stimulates
Blood and
Qi)

Sp6 (stimulates
Blood and
Qi)

Ki6 (assists
Ki Qi.
Also Yin Chiao)

Pe7 (regulates
the Qi)

116

with congestion in the chest, accompanied by lack of appetite and possible vomiting and diarrhoea. The pulse will be rapid and slippery, the tongue covered with a thick, greasy fur.

The spleen being the organ most notably at fault, treatment is directed to tonifying the spleen and removing the stagnation – CV12 (Zhongwan), St21 (Liangmen), St25 (Tianshu), St36 (Zusanli), Co4 (Hegu) and Bl20 (Pishu) spring readily to mind.

Traditional causes also include Blood Stagnation and Blood Deficiency.

## Blood Stagnation

This has the usual abdominal pain worse for pressure, scanty lochia with dark clots, a continuous fever, wiry and retarded pulse and a purplish tongue. Points previously cited for this condition are used: CV4 (Guanyuan), Sp6 (Sanyinjiao), Sp10 (Xuehai), Co11 (Quchi), Li3 (Taichong) and Bl32 (Ciliao) etc.

## Deficiency of Blood

This is due to blood loss during the delivery. It is a low-grade fever, but accompanied by excessive perspiration and often dizziness and palpitations. The patient will feel thirsty, and may have numbness in the hands and feet. The pulse will be big and hollow, the tongue pale with little or no fur. Alternatively, there may be a tidal or alternating fever and chills, with an aversion to cold, and pallor, vertigo, and constipation. The patient will feel tired, with a weakness in the low back and knees. The pulse will now be weak and thready, the tongue pale with no fur.

In both cases the principle is the same – tonify the Qi and Blood, via Bl20 (Pishu), Bl23 (Shenshu), Bl38 (Gaohuangshu), Sp6 (Sanyinjiao), St36 (Zusanlu), Ki6 (Zhaohai) and P7 (Daling).

Fevers due to cerebro-vascular accidents are also described, but the treatment of these is outside the scope of this particular book, and the reader is referred to the author's *Acupuncture Treatment of Musculo-Skeletal Conditions* for a full description.

# CONSTIPATION

Constipation after delivery is a very common condition and is due to the consequential loss of body fluids, leading to 'drying up' of the stools and intestines. As the strain of labour can also produce a Yin deficiency, this in its turn can lead to a 'false fire' causing a still greater evaporation of the fluids.

The simple loss of body fluids is treated as a deficiency of blood, and apart from the constipation the patient will have a dry, sallow complexion, normal appetite, and no abdominal swelling. The pulse will be weak and slow, the tongue light red.

Where there is a concomitant deficiency of Yin with False Fire, the abdomen will be distended and painful, the urine concentrated, the patient will be thirsty, and there may even be fever. Here, the pulse may be either thready and hesitant or deep and forceful, depending upon the amount of reaction by the body, and the tongue will be redder and develop a sticky yellow fur.

In both cases we must nourish the blood and promote the fluids, with points such as Bl20 (Pishu), St36 (Zusanli), Bl17 (Geshu) and Bl38 (Gaohuangshu), but in the latter instance we also use points to remove the heat – Sp10 (Xuehai) and Ki6 (Zhaohai). The point St25 (Tianshu) will stimulate the flow of blood and Qi and, as the Mu point of the Colon, will also have a specific effect upon the bowels, whilst TH6 (Zhigou) removes stagnation, particularly in the bowels.

# CONSTIPATION

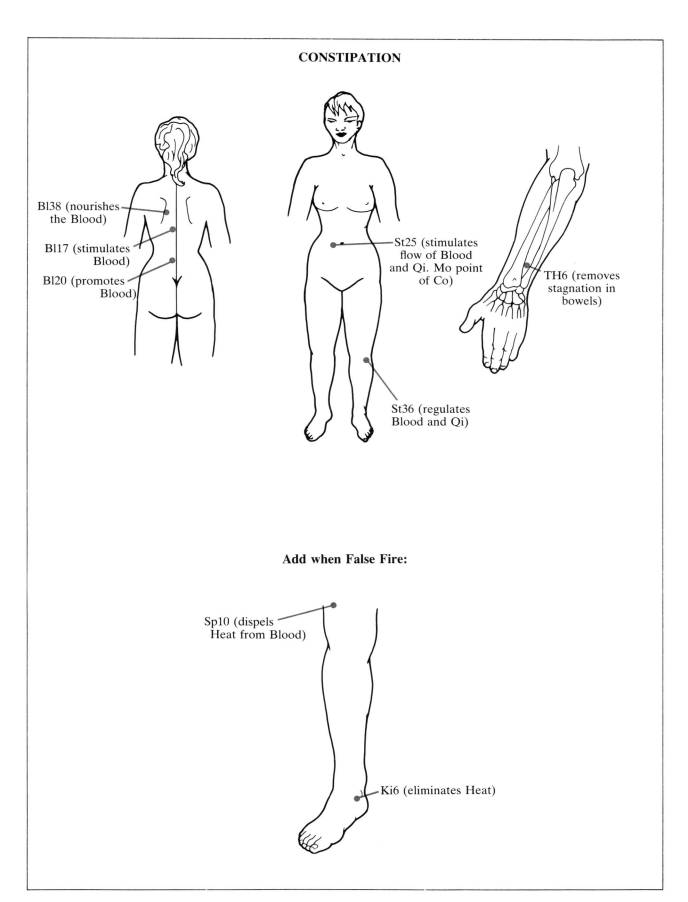

Bl38 (nourishes the Blood)

Bl17 (stimulates Blood)

Bl20 (promotes Blood)

St25 (stimulates flow of Blood and Qi. Mo point of Co)

St36 (regulates Blood and Qi)

TH6 (removes stagnation in bowels)

**Add when False Fire:**

Sp10 (dispels Heat from Blood)

Ki6 (eliminates Heat)

# URINARY INCONTINENCE

The general weakness of Qi after delivery can affect the kidneys and lead to incontinence. The basic deficiency of Qi presents as either polyuria or incontinence, with the passing of clear urine. The patient will be generally weak and tired, with a hollow pulse and a pale tongue. To stimulate the Qi the usual points are used: CV3 (Zhongji) – which will also have a specific effect as the Mo point of the Bladder – CV4 (Guanyuan), CV6 (Qihai), St36 (Zusanli), St25 (Tianshu) etc.

If the kidneys also become affected the complexion will assume a darker hue, and the usual weakness of the low back and knees associated with kidney deficiency will appear. The pulse will become deeper and the tongue moister. To such points as the above we can add those for kidney deficiency, e.g. GV4 (Mingmen), Bl23 (Shenshu), Ki3 (Taixi), Sp6 (Sanyinjiao) and others.

# URINARY INCONTINENCE
## To stimulate Qi:

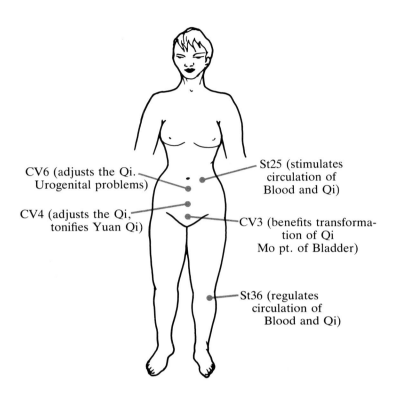

CV6 (adjusts the Qi.
Urogenital problems)

St25 (stimulates
circulation of
Blood and Qi)

CV4 (adjusts the Qi,
tonifies Yuan Qi)

CV3 (benefits transforma-
tion of Qi
Mo pt. of Bladder)

St36 (regulates
circulation of
Blood and Qi)

## When Kidney deficiency, add:

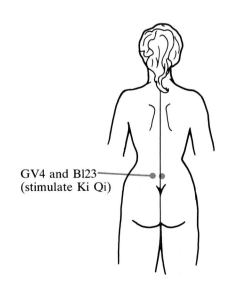

GV4 and Bl23
(stimulate Ki Qi)

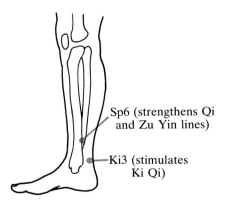

Sp6 (strengthens Qi
and Zu Yin lines)

Ki3 (stimulates
Ki Qi)

# SCANTY LACTATION

Whilst the Stomach component of the Yang Ming is important for its local effect, the Jue Yin irrigates the nipple and the Liver component of this is responsible for the movement of blood and Qi.

Traditionally, it is regarded that the milk is produced by the Qi and Blood in Chong Mai and Ren Mai. Insufficiency of milk, or lack of flow, is dependent upon one of two factors:

## (a) A weakness of Qi and a lack of Blood

This is due to a poor physical condition produced by either the strain of child-bearing and/or malnutrition and will cause scanty or no lactation at all. It is characterized by the fact that the breasts are small and flaccid, with no pain. The patient exhibits the usual pallor and fatigue, possibly blurred vision, dizziness, tinnitus, palpitations and lack of appetite, with heat in the palms and soles. There may be watery stools alternating with constipation. The pulse is thready and weak and the tongue pale.

It is a Xu condition, so reinforcement is required. Moxa CV17 (Shanzhong), and St18 (Rugen) – both points to stimulate the Qi and also to have a local effect – and needle Bl20 (Pishu), St36 (Zusanli), and SI1 (Shaoze). This latter point is an empirical point for affecting lactation. Bl17 (Geshu) and Bl18 (Ganshu) may also be thought of.

## (b) Stagnant Liver Qi

This is often regarded as due to emotional causes such as anger, frustration or depression. It will depress the liver or spleen and, by preventing the free movement, cause an accumulation of stuck Qi and blood in the breasts, which become distended, full and painful. The patient may also have a feeling of oppression in the chest, with eructation (possibly hiccups), nausea, pains in the sides, and a feeling of pressure in the head leading to headaches. The pulse is wiry and retarded, the tongue has a thin, white, greasy fur.

It is a Shi condition, but the stagnation needs moving, so once again moxa CV17 (Shanzhong) and St18 (Rugen), but this time follow by reducing SI1 (Shaoze), Li14 (Qimen) and P6 (Neiguan).

This condition can show the presence of lumps in the breast which may eventually lead to mastitis.

# SCANTY LACTATION

## Weakness of Qi

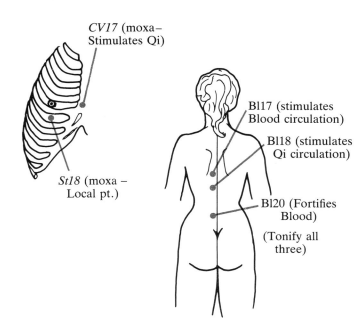

*CV17* (moxa–
Stimulates Qi)

*St18* (moxa –
Local pt.)

Bl17 (stimulates
Blood circulation)

Bl18 (stimulates
Qi circulation)

Bl20 (Fortifies
Blood)

(Tonify all
three)

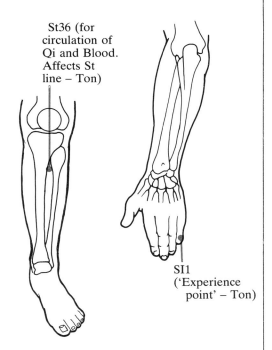

St36 (for
circulation of
Qi and Blood.
Affects St
line – Ton)

SI1
('Experience
point' – Ton)

## Stagnant Liver Qi

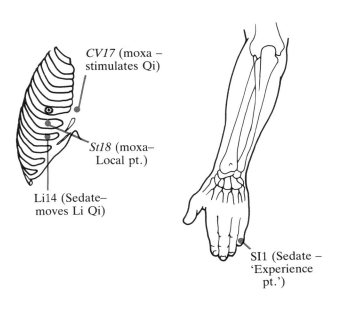

*CV17* (moxa –
stimulates Qi)

*St18* (moxa–
Local pt.)

Li14 (Sedate–
moves Li Qi)

SI1 (Sedate –
'Experience
pt.')

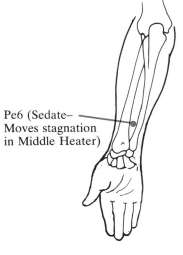

Pe6 (Sedate–
Moves stagnation
in Middle Heater)

# MASTITIS

This condition is frequently caused by an infection of one or more segments of the breast from the entry of bacteria along a duct or through a cracked nipple. If severe, an abcess may form. The breast becomes swollen and painful and an area of redness may be seen, more usually on the under-surface of the breast. It is more often than not accompanied by a rise in temperature. If an abcess is formed, surgical intervention is possibly recommended.

Where infection is not the causative factor, other factors may be improper suckling, where the infant 'blows' at the breast, over-indulgence in fatty foods or from emotional disturbances – this latter results in the stagnation of Liver Qi which was dealt with in the preceding section.

As with scanty lactation, a deficiency of Qi and blood could predispose to the development of mastitis. The overall general deficiency symptoms will be the same, but the inflammation in the breast tissues wil produce pain with hard, rock-like indurations.

The general treatment is the same – moxa CV17 (Shanzhong) and St18 (Rugen), possibly adding Sp18 (Tianxi) for stronger effect, and needle Bl20 (Pishu), St36 (Zusanli) and SI1 (Shaoze), adding Sp6 (Sanyinjiao) for its effect on the Zu Jue Yin.

In the more usual type of mastitis due to infection, the breast will demonstrate the typical signs of inflammation of heat, redness, pain and swelling, worse for any pressure and, because of the general effect upon the body as a whole, fever with no perspiration, headache, and pains in all the joints. The pulse will be superficial and tight or rapid. Treatment in this stage is designed more for its local anti-inflammatory effect – St18 (Rugen), St34 (Liangqiu), SI1 (Shaoze) and Co4 (Hegu) to affect the local Yang Ming, and GB20 (Feng-chi) to eliminate internal wind and because of its effect upon the liver (Zu Jue Yin).

As the condition worsens into suppuration the breast tissues become more 'soggy' and the redness of the inflammation spreads over the whole breast, with intense throbbing pain. The pulse becomes fuller and the tongue develops a yellow fur. Treatment now must be on a deeper level, with points such as Co11 (Quchi), Bl54 (Weizhong), P6 (Neiguan), GB21 (Jianjing), Li3 (Taichong) and St36 (Zusanli). It is only fair to state that the author's considered opinion is that in the case of a specific bacterial infection the use of antibiotics is to be preferred, and acupuncture resorted to only where the patient has a definite allergy to their employment. Acupuncture can be used to support the patient's general health and well-being.

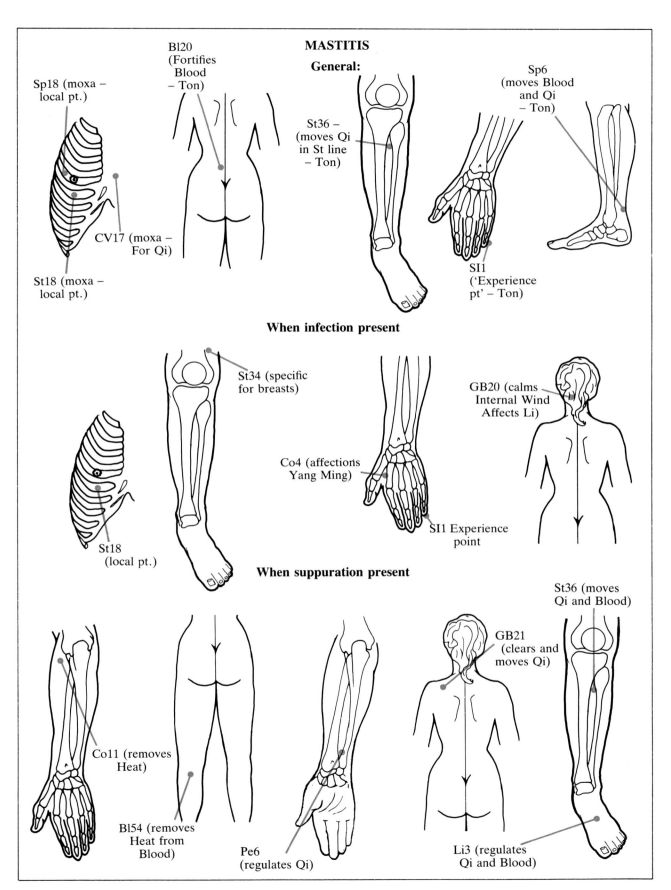

# MASTITIS

**General:**

Sp18 (moxa –
local pt.)

Bl20
(Fortifies
Blood
– Ton)

Sp6
(moves Blood
and Qi
– Ton)

St36 –
(moves Qi
in St line
– Ton)

CV17 (moxa –
For Qi)

St18 (moxa –
local pt.)

SI1
('Experience
pt' – Ton)

**When infection present**

St34 (specific
for breasts)

GB20 (calms
Internal Wind
Affects Li)

Co4 (affections
Yang Ming)

St18
(local pt.)

SI1 Experience
point

**When suppuration present**

St36 (moves
Qi and Blood)

GB21
(clears and
moves Qi)

Co11 (removes
Heat)

Bl54 (removes
Heat from
Blood)

Pe6
(regulates Qi)

Li3 (regulates
Qi and Blood)

# SUMMARY

As a last general summary:

Menses earlier than usual – may signify Heat causing reckless movement of blood, or that Deficient Qi cannot govern the blood. It is differentiated by the accompanying signs: Red tongue = Heat, pale tongue = Deficient Qi.

Late periods suggest Deficient Blood or Cold causing stagnation.

Irregular menses are often a sign that Liver Qi is not moving harmoniously.

Excess flow may signify Heat in the Blood, or Deficient Qi.

Insufficient flow or lack of menses may mean Deficient Blood, Cold obstructing the Blood, or Congealed Blood.

Pale and thin menstrual blood points to a deficient condition.

Bright red blood suggests Heat.

Very dark blood also suggests Heat, and blood that is purplish, especially if clotted, may indicate Congealed or Stagnated Blood.

Copious, clear or white, and thin discharges (leucorrhoea) usually signify deficiency and Dampness.

Discharges which are thick and yellow, or accompanied by itching or soreness of the vagina, are often signs of Heat and Dampness.

Generally: Pain *before* a period is due to Stagnation of Qi

*during* is due to Stagnation of Blood

*after* is due to deficient Blood and Qi

From an inability to leave well alone;
From too much zeal for what is new and contempt for what is old;
From putting knowledge before wisdom, science before art, cleverness before common-sense,
From treating patients as cases; and
From making the cure of a disease more grievous than its endurance,
Good Lord, deliver us.
– Sir Robert Hutchinson (1871–1960)

# INDEX

(Figures in *italics* refer to illustrations)